# Paedia
# Clinic
# Examinations
## Second Edition

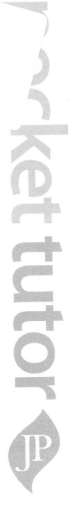

# Paediatric Clinical Examination
## Second Edition

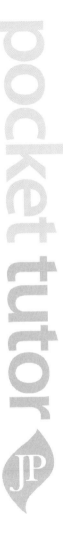

**Keir Shiels** MA MB BChir MRCPCH MAcadMEd
Specialty Registrar in Paediatrics
Royal London Hospital
Barts Health NHS Trust
London, UK

**Rossa Brugha** BMBCh MA(Oxon) MRCPCH PhD
Consultant Respiratory Paediatrician
King's College Hospital NHS Foundation Trust
London, UK

JP
medical
publishers

© 2020 Jaypee Brothers Medical Publishers

First edition 2013

Published by Jaypee Brothers Medical Publishers,
4838/24 Ansari Road, New Delhi, India

Tel: +91 (011) 43574357              Fax: +91 (011)43574390

Email: info@jpmedpub.com, jaypee@jaypeebrothers.com
Web: www.jpmedpub.com, www.jaypeebrothers.com

JPM is the imprint of Jaypee Brothers Medical Publishers.

ISBN: 978-1-909836-89-1

**British Library Cataloguing in Publication Data**
A catalogue record for this book is available from the British Library

**Library of Congress Cataloging in Publication Data**
A catalog record for this book is available from the Library of Congress

| | |
|---|---|
| Development Editor: | Harsha Madan |
| Editorial Assistant: | Keshav Kumar |
| Cover Design: | Rakesh Kumar |

# Foreword

The history and examination of a child remains the cornerstone of paediatrics. Initially, it appears to be a daunting task. Children range in age, from newborn infants to young adults, and the medical conditions encountered vary markedly with age. They often do not wish to be examined, so the examiner needs to know exactly what information they are seeking and how to persuade the child to allow them obtain it.

In *Pocket Tutor Paediatric Clinical Examination*, Keir Shiels and Rossa Brugha expertly guide you through dealing with these problems. Starting with a brief general introduction to history and examination in children, common presentations and examination for each system of the body are then described. There are also case scenarios which demonstrate how they relate to clinical practice, and Clinical Insight boxes explaining how the examination or pathology differs from adult medicine. New to this edition are numerous photographs demonstrating examination techniques and showing the clinical conditions described.

All this information is succinctly condensed into a highly readable, pocket-sized book. It is an invaluable guide to the clinical examination of children, and the authors have admirably succeeded in their aim to provide a structured approach to examining children that is both stimulating and informative.

**Tom Lissauer**
Honorary Consultant Paediatrician
Imperial College Healthcare Trust
May 2019

# Preface

Working with children is one of the most rewarding and enjoyable experiences you will have in medicine. But it isn't easy. Children are not little adults: you will have to contend with patients of very differing sizes, abilities and levels of understanding.

In writing the second edition of *Pocket Tutor Paediatric Clinical Examination*, we have kept the original approach within each chapter: common presentations followed by a structured examination. Within this framework, however, much has changed. New Clinical Insight boxes provide tips on how paediatric examination or pathology differs from adult medicine, and each chapter now has a summary table. Examinations that are unique to children have been expanded: auxology and pubertal staging are now covered in more detail. By combining some chapters (ENT and neck lumps, for example), we have made more room for figures and tables. There is a new chapter on children's behaviour, and an expanded section on multisystem syndromes.

While paediatricians do occasionally have to deal with harrowing and exceptionally difficult situations, these are fortunately rare. Paediatrics is surely one of the most rewarding medical specialties and it is certainly one of the broadest. We hope this book whets your appetite for it.

**Keir Shiels**
**Rossa Brugha**
May 2019

# Contents

# Acknowledgements

This book would not have been possible without the support and participation of many kind and generous people. Thank you in particular to my friend and colleague Rossa Brugha, who started me on this journey with an excellent first edition, words of advice and a personal recommendation to the publishers. Tom Banister-Fletcher and Adam Rajah of JP Medical have provided sterling support by polishing, tweaking and editing this project from manuscript to book.

But the real heroes of this endeavour have been those who have sacrificed their time – and their dignity – to sit patiently for hours having their photographs taken. Thank you to Dr Kate Sullivan, the Sinnett family, the Van-der-Velde family and the Douieb family for travelling to be photographed.

To the patients and parents who happily gave their consent for their illnesses to be used in this book, at a time of angst and concern, I – and many future paediatricians – will be eternally grateful. To charities who helped source photographs – particularly the Turner Syndrome Society and the Max Appeal – thank you for your time, your patience and your tuition: you have taught me more in email correspondence than I ever learned in lectures or clinic. Your lessons will stay with me.

Thank you also the Down Syndrome Medical Interest Group for granting permission to use Figure 4.5, and to the Royal College of Paediatricians for Figure 4.4.

But my biggest thanks must go to my partner Peter Amies, whose diligence, willing self-sacrifice and patience, at incredibly short notice, have been abused in the taking, selecting and editing of the new pictures in this edition. You are a gem: and I am incredibly lucky.

Figure 6.2, 7.1 and 9.1 are reproduced from Cartledge P et al. Pocket Tutor Clinical Examination Second Edition. London: JP Medical, 2019.

# History taking

History taking in paediatrics differs in many ways from history taking in adult medicine. Extra areas to ask about include perinatal history, immunisations and developmental milestones. As babies and young children cannot speak for themselves, history taking becomes a three-way process involving the child, the health-care staff, and the parents or carers. Well-developed communication skills are a vital attribute for a paediatrician.

## 1.1 Clinical scenario

### A baby in respiratory distress

A father brings a 9-month-old girl into the paediatric emergency department because she has a runny nose, has suddenly started coughing and is short of breath. These are all signs of a respiratory infection (see **Chapter 6**).

#### Differential diagnosis

The differential diagnosis includes:

- bronchiolitis
- virus-induced wheeze
- pneumonia
- pneumonitis
- pertussis

#### Further information

The father says that his daughter has had a mild cold for 3 days but no fever. She had been well and playing happily until about 2 hours ago when he came back into the living room after making a cup of tea and saw she had suddenly become very short of breath.

The baby is fully vaccinated and developing normally. She can pick up small objects in a pincer grip and enjoys putting things in her mouth.

When the father is asked what she had been playing with, he says that she was playing with her brother's small building bricks.

## Conclusion

A good history prompts reconsideration of prior assumptions. The sudden onset of respiratory distress changes the differential diagnosis from respiratory infection to:
- pneumothorax
- inhaled foreign body

Suspicion of the latter yields results in this case: a chest radiograph shows a building brick in the right main bronchus.

# 1.2 Preparation

Ensure you have as much key relevant information as possible rather than just the notes for the most recent clerking. This can be obtained from multiple sources. For example, if a child is known to have a history of family neglect, information may be found on the Child Protection Register and with social services. Nurseries, schools, midwives, health visitors and GPs are other sources.

Triage notes and referral letters contain, for example, a brief summary of the presenting problem, physiological observations and some social history. However, make sure you approach each case freshly, so that any documented history does not unduly influence how you collect information in the current clinical encounter. An illness may also have evolved since the most recent correspondence.

## Setting up

Pay attention to the surroundings:
- Close the door or curtain to maintain confidentiality.
- Avoid obstacles, e.g. a desk, between you and the family.
- Ensure that everyone including the child has a place to sit.
- Aim to be on a similar eye level to the child.
- Ensure distractions are available for younger children, e.g. toys and videos (see **Chapter 3**).

# 1.3 Communication

The complex dynamics of communication in paediatrics include:
- a direct history from the patient
- a vicarious history from the accompanying adult
- a contextual history from a referring GP or school
- a different approach with patients of different ages
- a repeated history in the absence of the accompanying adult

## Who am I talking to?

Most paediatric medicine involves children aged <5 years, so the history is usually taken from a parent. However, this approach is open to a number of challenges. For example, some older children have a sound appreciation of their own health (sometimes very different from the parent's ideas).

Establish who has accompanied the child to hospital. Adults accompanying a child may include:
- parents
- grandparents, aunts and uncles
- older siblings
- nannies or babysitters
- teachers
- foster-parents
- social workers
- police, firefighters or paramedics
- neighbours
- interpreters
- religious/community leaders

### Clinical insight

Instead of asking the accompanying adult who they are, ask the child who they have brought to hospital with them. This keeps the child at the centre of the consultation. Confirm with the adult what they would like to be called. Many parents prefer to be addressed by their name, rather than 'Mum' or 'Dad'.

Many family units do not fit with the traditional family model. Be sensitive to the fact that a child may be being brought up by a same-sex couple.

Establishing who is accompanying the child is more than simple courtesy. Throughout this book, the word 'parent' is often used to mean 'accompanying adult'. However, bear in mind that, regardless of who accompanies the child, only a parent or legal guardian can provide legal consent for procedures, operations and intimate examinations.

## Language

Check whether the individuals involved in the consultation speak the same language as you. Interpreting is a difficult skill. Be aware that family members acting as interpreters may have conflicting views or may try to help by directly answering questions that are intended for somebody else. An impartial professional interpreter (in person or on the phone) is the gold standard. 'In your own words' is a useful phrase to use.

Modify your language according to the age of the child. Do not patronise an adolescent or confuse a child with jargon.

Be aware that young children may not have a precise or accurate vocabulary. A 4-year-old complaining of pain in the 'neck' is just as likely to be describing pain in the throat. Young children may complain of 'headache' or 'tummy pain' as a way of articulating a general feeling of illness.

### Clinical insight

A technique that allows you to spend a suitably long time observing a baby while maintaining conversation with the parents is to address your questions directly to the baby. This often feels silly, but the parents will answer.

### Active observation

Remember to look at the child while you are taking the history. For example, if a child with 'awful tummy pain' is running around, the pain is at least sporadic and may be constipation rather than appendicitis.

Approaching a shy young child can make them cry, which makes the examination far more challenging. There are techniques to deal with this (see **Chapters 2** and **3**). Use the window of opportunity afforded by history taking to look from a distance for clinical signs such as lethargy, respiratory distress and cyanosis.

# 1.4 Components of the paediatric history

The components of a paediatric history are:
- name and date of birth
- name of accompanying adult and relationship
- age (adjusted for prematurity if necessary)
- weight and height
- presenting complaint
- history of presenting complaint
- past medical, drug and allergy history
- antenatal, birth and developmental history
- immunisation history
- family and social history
- systems review

## Presenting complaint

The presenting complaint is a symptom or sign that has caused the parents or child to seek medical attention. This may be something:
- easily observed (e.g. respiratory distress)
- intermittent (e.g. a fever)
- harder to spot at first glance (e.g. reduced feeding)
- very nebulous (e.g. 'just not being himself')

Each of the four examples above could be a presentation of bronchiolitis but different parents will be most concerned about different aspects of the condition based on their experience, culture and support network.

Start with an open question such as, 'What is the problem?' or 'How can I help?'

## History of the presenting complaint

Use the **TENDS** mnemonic to structure the history:
- **Triggers** – does anything cause it to associate/worsen/improve?
- **Evolution** – how has the symptom changed over time? Does it come and go?

- **Nature** – how does it manifest or feel? Does it move or radiate anywhere?
- **Duration** – how long has it gone on for? Is it constant or intermittent?
- **Severity** – can it be rated on a scale or quantified? How worrying is it for the child or parent?

The **TENDS** mnemonic allows a differential diagnosis to be whittled down. For example, vomiting that is **T**riggered by coughing, and has a short **D**uration and variable **S**everity from a couple of teaspoons to a whole feed, is likely to be bronchiolitis (see page 87) or pneumonia (see page 89). Vomiting **T**riggered by feeding with a few weeks' **D**uration of worsening and a **S**everity that is now projectile vomiting of whole feeds is more likely to be pyloric stenosis (see page 131).

## Past medical history

Enquire about previous illnesses, hospital admissions and operations. Note whether the child was born prematurely (see page 18).

## Drug and allergy history

This should cover:
- medications and allergies
- previous medications
- over-the-counter medications and dietary supplements that the child is taking

Clarify the dose the child is taking: parents often quote the dose of syrups in millilitres rather than milligrams.

As some medications can be used for more than one indication, document why a child is taking a particular drug. Beta-blockers, for example, can be used in the treatment of hypertension, migraine or anxiety.

## Paediatric extras

A paediatric history also includes:
- antenatal history
- birth history

- developmental history
- immunisation history

The level of detail required depends on the context. For example, it is vital to elicit a detailed perinatal history for a child who has a developmental problem but less important for an adolescent with asthma.

## Antenatal history

The antenatal history should cover:
- whether the pregnancy was planned or unplanned
- whether the conception was natural or, e.g. involved in vitro fertilisation or donor eggs
- the results of antenatal ultrasound
- drugs used by the mother and illnesses that occurred during pregnancy
- the mother's blood group

Antenatal complications can have repercussions on the developing fetus (see **Chapter 2**).

## Birth history

Make a note of:
- the type of delivery – spontaneous, induced, instrumental or caesarean?
- the reasons for a caesarean delivery
- complications surrounding the birth
- Apgar scores (see **Chapter 2**)
- birthweight
- admissions to the neonatal intensive care unit
- treatment that was required in the postnatal ward

## Developmental history

Delayed milestones or regression should be recorded (see **Chapter 5**).

## Immunisations

Most countries have a national schedule for immunisation, but these also vary on a local level. For example, the BCG vaccine (against tuberculosis) is given at birth in some, but not all, areas of London based on local prevalence of tuberculosis. Some vaccines are offered on a more individualised basis – for example, in the UK, typhoid vaccine is only given to individuals who are travelling to designated at-risk countries.

**Table 1.1** shows the vaccination schedule for children in the UK at the time of publication.

**Controversies** You need to be able to have an informed discussion with children, parents and families about immunisation because there has been conflicting and misleading media coverage of its safety. This particularly relates to:
- a postulated link between the measles, mumps and rubella (MMR) vaccine and autism
- the contents of vaccines being toxic
- vaccination when young 'overloading' the immune system

None of these claims has held up to scientific scrutiny. Countries no longer using the MMR vaccine, such as Japan, have seen no change in incidence of autism.

| Age | Vaccine* |
|---|---|
| 8 weeks | 6-in-1, pneumococcal, Men B, rotavirus |
| 12 weeks | 6-in-1, rotavirus |
| 16 weeks | 6-in-1, pneumococcal, Men B |
| 1 year | HiB/Men C, MMR, pneumococcal, Men B |
| 3 years 4 months | MMR, 4-in-1 |
| 2–9 years annually | Influenza |
| 12 years (girls only) | Human papillomavirus (cervical cancer) |
| 14 years | Men ACWY, 3-in-1 |

*6-in-1, diphtheria, tetanus, pertussis, *Haemophilus influenzae* B (HiB), hepatitis B and polio combined in one injection. 4-in-1, diphtheria, tetanus, pertussis and polio combined in one injection. 3-in-1, diphtheria, tetanus and polio. MMR, measles, mumps and rubella combined in one injection.
Men, meningococcal disease.

**Table 1.1** The UK vaccination schedule (2018). Always check national resources for updates

Be aware that families may have opinions contrary to your own. Focus on establishing the child's vaccination status, and forming a differential diagnosis.

## Family and social history

Children have two core social units: the family, and school or nursery. A good opening question is, 'Who lives at home?' Ask about school, nursery, childcare and relationships, including whether the child's parents are still in a relationship with each other.

Ask about major illnesses in the family and whether the mother has a history of recurrent miscarriages. Bear in mind some conditions that run in families may be adult-onset 'red herrings': explore what parents mean by, for example, 'diabetes' or 'heart disease'. Ask about consanguinity in the parents.

It often helps to draw a family tree, going back two generations. **Figure 1.1** shows the symbols that are used. A family tree enables you to trace a genetic illness to establish heritability, as

> ## Clinical insight
>
> Adolescents may have a more complex social history than their parents realise. Ask about mental health, sex, relationships, bullying, drugs, alcohol and social media. This is best done with the parents out of the room and a chaperone present. Do not miss an ectopic pregnancy just because an adolescent denies being sexually active when her parents are present.

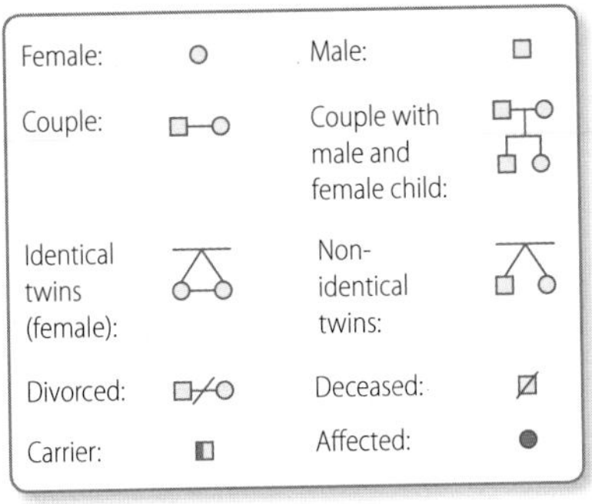

| | | | |
|---|---|---|---|
| Female: | ○ | Male: | □ |
| Couple: | □—○ | Couple with male and female child: | |
| Identical twins (female): | | Non-identical twins: | |
| Divorced: | □/○ | Deceased: | |
| Carrier: | ▣ | Affected: | ● |

**Figure 1.1** Symbols used when constructing a family tree.

well as to work out who is who in a complex social setting. Ask whether other children in school or nursery have been ill, and how long the child has been attending. Children are exposed to multiple infections in the first few months at nursery.

## Systems review

These questions allow you to ask about the function of organ systems that the parent believes are only tangentially related to the presenting problem. Significant clues can be found, such as constipation in hypothyroidism, or obstructive sleep apnoea in a hyperactive child. Ask about:

- growth, feeding, diet (see **Chapter 4**)
- respiratory or cardiac problems (see **Chapters 6** and **7**)
- bowel and bladder habit (see **Chapter 8**)
- headaches, fits and 'funny turns' (see **Chapter 9**)
- exercise
- fever and rashes (see **Chapter 12**)
- concentration, sleep and social interaction (see **Chapter 13**)

If the child is of an appropriate age, ask about school and whether the symptoms are equally apparent in the classroom and at home.

## Summary and questions

Summarise to the child and parents what they have just told you. This gives you a chance to go back over their concerns if they feel something has been missed.

Follow this summary by giving the opportunity to ask questions. People may not ask direct questions unless they are invited to.

## 1.5 Red flags

'Red flag' symptoms or signs are suggestive of serious pathology and must be managed with advice from senior medical and nursing staff. **Table 1.2** contains a list of red flags symptoms that the history can uncover.

Children are not little adults. Symptoms that are red flags in adult medicine may not carry the same level of concern in

| Red flag | Possible diagnosis |
|---|---|
| Headache waking child at night Nocturnal vomiting | Brain tumour |
| Fracture in non-ambulant child | Non-accidental injury |
| Green vomit | Bowel obstruction |
| Fever in a child <4 months old | Sepsis |
| Limp without a history of trauma | Sepsis, malignancy |
| Weight loss | Diabetes, malignancy, inflammatory bowel disease |
| Non-blanching rash | Sepsis, idiopathic thrombocytopoenic purpura, haemolytic uraemic syndrome, leukaemia, haemophilia |
| Anuria | Renal failure |
| Irritable baby/acute behavioural change | Meningitis, encephalitis |

Table 1.2  Red flags symptoms in the history

paediatrics. For example, it is very unlikely that central chest pain is a myocardial infarction in a 5-year-old – gastric reflux is more likely. Similarly, an apparently innocuous symptom such a limp, which may be of little concern in an adult, can be a sign of malignancy in a child.

Red flags from the examination are discussed in **Chapter 3**.

# The newborn

Examination of the newborn baby is a screening process that examines every organ system. Congenital abnormalities may need to be swiftly dealt with, so newborns are examined by a healthcare professional at least three times in the first minutes, days and weeks of life, even if they seem well. The examination must always be put into the context of a full maternal and fetal history.

## At delivery

The Apgar score (**Table 2.1**) is calculated at 1, 5 and 10 minutes after birth. It is a simple indicator of the need to escalate resuscitation. The lower the Apgar score at 5 and 10 minutes, the higher the likelihood of poor long-term neurological development. If resuscitation is not required, a general inspection is carried out at this point for anatomical abnormalities, such as ambiguous genitalia and omphalocoele.

| Feature | Score = 0 | Score = 1 | Score = 2 |
|---|---|---|---|
| Appearance | White | Blue | Pink |
| Pulse | No heart rate | <100 beats per minute | >100 beats per minute |
| Grimace to stimulation | No response | Weak grimace or feeble cry | Good cry, flexed tone |
| Activity | None, floppy | Some flexion | Actively flexed |
| Respiration | Not breathing | Weak, irregular, gasps | Good cry or regular respirations |

Score the baby out of 2 for each feature. Aggregate the scores to reach a total (maximum 10).

Table 2.1 Apgar score

### Formal neonatal check

Colloquially known as the 'baby check', this detailed examination must be performed no earlier than 6 hours of life. This gives the fetal circulation time to adapt, thus avoiding false-positive results such as heart murmurs (see page 107) and mottled skin (see page 19).

### At 6–8 weeks

The examination is repeated to ensure the child is growing and feeding well. It may also uncover problems that, for physiological reasons, were not apparent in the first few days of life. These include the murmur of a left-to-right shunt caused by a ventricular septal defect (see page 108).

## 2.1 Clinical scenario

### A neonate with a rash

A midwife is concerned about a rash on a newborn baby. The baby seems well despite the florid rash on the trunk and back. There are multiple small, tense, bright yellow spots with red halos around them.

### Differential diagnosis

The following diagnoses should be considered:
- erythema toxicum
- pustulosis
- folliculitis
- sepsis

### Further information

The spots are not easily burst. There are no risk factors for sepsis in the maternal history, and examination is otherwise normal. The baby is happy and feeding well.

### Conclusion

Because the baby is well, and the appearance and distribution of the rash is typical of erythema toxicum (see page 24), the rash will resolve spontaneously.

## A neonate with jaundice

A 3-day-old baby, born by caesarean section at term, is brought to the emergency department with jaundice that was spotted by the community midwife. The baby has been crying a lot and struggling to latch on during feeding. His skin and sclerae are visibly yellow. The anterior fontanelle is sunken and his weight is 10% lower than his birthweight.

### Differential diagnosis

The differential diagnosis includes:
- poor feeding and dehydration
- breast-milk jaundice
- blood group incompatibility
- sepsis
- conjugated jaundice

### Further information

There are no antenatal risk factors for sepsis. The stool is seedy and yellow, and the urine clear. The liver is not palpable. The bilirubin level is elevated and is plotted on a term neonate jaundice chart. Blood tests show a normal fraction of conjugated bilirubin, and no anaemia. The rest of the examination is normal.

### Conclusion

Because the baby is otherwise well, the diagnosis is jaundice secondary to poor feeding. The baby is admitted to the postnatal ward for phototherapy and feeding support.

## 2.2 Maternal history

Check for all maternal factors that can cause illness in the neonate (**Table 2.2**). Review serology results and immunity screens for congenital infections, and take a vaccination history.

Bear in mind that the fetus can be affected by conditions in the mother that:
- are present before pregnancy (e.g. systemic lupus erythematosus)

| Maternal condition | Effects on the baby |
|---|---|
| Diabetes mellitus | Macrosomia, hypoglycaemia, polycythaemia |
| Hyperthyroidism | Hypothyroidism or hyperthyroidism |
| Systemic lupus erythematosus | Congenital heart block |
| Congenital infections | Deafness (CMV, toxoplasmosis), sepsis (bacterial infections), HIV, encephalitis (HSV), hepatitis B |
| Infections during pregnancy | Developmental abnormalities (rubella, toxoplasmosis) blindness (CMV), microcephaly (Zika virus) |
| Teratogenic medications | Spina bifida, phocomelia, cardiac abnormalities |
| Pre-eclampsia | Intrauterine growth restriction |
| Smoking | Decreased birthweight, cleft palate, heart defects |
| Excess alcohol intake | Fetal alcohol syndrome |
| CMV, cytomegalovirus; HSV, herpes simplex virus. | |

**Table 2.2** Medical conditions in pregnancy and their effects on the newborn

- arise as a result of pregnancy (e.g. gestational diabetes)
- are a discrete episode during pregnancy (e.g. rubella infection)
- are asymptomatic (e.g. group B streptococcal colonisation)
- are treated with medication with known side effects (e.g. labetalol infusion for maternal hypertension resulting in neonatal hypoglycaemia)
- are the results of a previous antibody-mediated condition (e.g. Graves' disease)

A number of acquired maternal infections cause morbidity and mortality in the developing fetus. Some infections are congenital (i.e. the baby is born infected with the same pathogen that is infecting the mother, e.g. HIV, syphilis); others (e.g. rubella) affect the in utero development of the fetus. Some infections (e.g. toxoplasmosis and cyto-megalovirus) fall into both categories.

## Drugs

Medications and other substances taken by the mother can seriously affect the infant:

- Lithium (a mood stabiliser) can cause cardiac abnormalities

### Clinical insight

Many women with a history of Graves' disease have undergone thyroidectomy and therefore describe themselves as 'hypothyroid' or 'taking thyroxine'. Ascertain why the mother is currently hypothyroid, and whether she has ever been hyperthyroid. The thyroid-stimulating antibodies of Graves' disease persist after thyroidectomy and can cross the placenta, resulting in transient neonatal hyperthyroidism.

- Sodium valproate (an anticonvulsant) can cause damage to the developing brain and neural tube (see page 302)
- Medical or recreational use of opiates can result in neonatal abstinence syndrome
- Smoking decreases fetal birthweight
- Excessive intake of alcohol may result in fetal alcohol syndrome, which is characterised by dysmorphic features and impaired intelligence (see page 300)

## 2.3 Development and delivery

Check for concerns relating to the health of the fetus, such as threatened miscarriage, poor or asymmetrical growth, or breech position.

Look at reports from antenatal scans – were abnormalities identified? Check the results of any genetic testing carried out on the fetus, such as amniocentesis or chorionic villus sampling.

Look at the expected due date and calculate the baby's gestation. Prematurity is classified using the World Health Organization scale (**Table 2.3**).

### Clinical insight

Risk factors for sepsis in newborn babies include:

- premature labour (<37 weeks' gestation)
- prolonged rupture of membranes (>24 hours)
- maternal group B streptococcal colonisation (on a vaginal swab)
- maternal fever during labour
- foul-smelling liquor (chorioamnionitis)

| Gestational age at birth (weeks) | World Health Organization classification |
|---|---|
| 37–42 | Term baby |
| 34–36 | Late preterm |
| 32–34 | Moderate preterm |
| 28–32 | Very preterm |
| <28 | Extreme preterm |

Table 2.3 Classification of prematurity

## Labour and delivery

Check:

- for a history of fetal distress, e.g. an abnormal cardiotocograph (CTG) or meconium-stained liquor (from a stressed infant who has opened the bowels and passed meconium)
- whether the delivery was vaginal, instrumental (forceps or Ventouse suction assisted) or caesarean
- whether resuscitation of the newborn was required following birth
- the birthweight and head circumference
- risk factors for sepsis in the baby

**Clinical insight**

Some babies pass meconium (the first sticky green-black stool) in utero, and this can enter the airway. The meconium can then be aspirated during the baby's first breath and cause severe pulmonary inflammation. Oxygen, intubation or extracorporeal membrane oxygenation may be required to stabilise the baby.

## 2.4 Examination of the newborn

Next, ask about breast-feeding, and encourage it if appropriate. For contraindications to breastfeeding see Chapter 4 (Table 4.2). Babies should be feeding every 2–4 hours.

Ask whether the baby has passed urine and meconium. Babies should open their bowels within the first 24 hours, and failure to do so may be an indicator of anal atresia or Hirschprung's disease. If the baby is settled, listen to the heart sounds and examine the eyes first as these are particularly challenging examinations in a crying baby.

## General inspection

### Colour

Check the baby's colour, which can indicate significant pathology (**Table 2.4**).

### Appearance

Does the baby look dysmorphic (i.e. have an abnormal facial appearance suggestive of a genetic abnormality – see **Chapter 14**)? Remember that in the first few days the

## Clinical insight

Jaundice is expected in babies because all neonates must break down the old fetal haemoglobin. This results in escalating bilirubin levels over the first 5 days of life. However, jaundice should not be visible within the first 24 hours, so a visibly jaundiced baby who is less than a day old must be thoroughly investigated and treated for possible sepsis.

Serum bilirubin level should be plotted on a gestational-age-appropriate jaundice chart for all jaundiced babies.

Jaundice may be easier to see in the eyes than the skin, especially in dark-skinned babies.

| Colour | Medical term | Pathology |
|---|---|---|
| Pink | Normal | Normal |
| Red | Plethora | Polycythaemia |
| Yellow | Jaundice | Blood group incompatibility, liver pathology, dehydration, breast milk associated |
| Blue | Cyanosis | Congenital cardiac disease, respiratory distress |
| White | Pallor | Blood loss |
| Grey | Grey baby | Sepsis, heart failure |
| Purple speckled face | Facial congestion | Difficult delivery |
| Purple speckled body, possibly with petechiae | Petechiae or purpura | Thrombocytopenia, clotting abnormality |
| Marble-like patterning of the skin | Mottling | Poor peripheral perfusion, sepsis, cardiac disease, hypothermia |

Table 2.4 Skin colours indicative of pathology

face may appear swollen as a result of oedema caused by the delivery.

If the child is awake, observe the muscle tone and movements (**Figure 2.1**).

## Skull

Note the following:

- overlapping sutures
- the anterior fontanelle (bulging, pulsatile, sunken or flat?)
- head shape (checking for fused or overlying sutures)
- cephalhaematoma (bleeding between the skull bone and periosteum)
- a subgaleal bleed (bleeding between the periosteum and the aponeurosis)
- occipitofrontal head circumference (**Figure 2.2**)

## Ears

Look for pits (small holes) and tags (small protrusions of extra skin) anterior to the tragus. These may be indicators of abnormal inner ear architecture and therefore prompt extra screening of hearing. Low-set ears are seen in some genetic conditions, including Down's syndrome (see page 287).

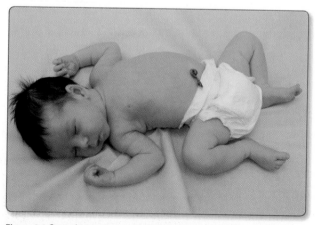

**Figure 2.1** General inspection: normal flexed tone in a neonate.

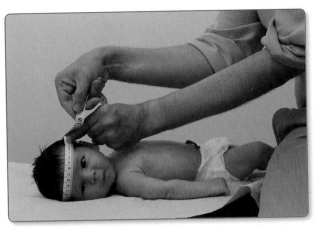

**Figure 2.2** Measuring the occipitofrontal circumference.

## Eyes

From a distance, elicit the red reflex in each eye using an ophthalmoscope (**Figure 2.3**). A child with leucocoria (**Figure 2.3b**), in which the pupil appears white, may have a cataract or congenital retinoblastoma and should be urgently referred to an ophthalmologist.

## Nose and mouth

- Check for patent nares or choanal atresia (in which one or both nostrils are occluded by bone). Babies are obligate nasal breathers so a baby with a blocked nostril struggles to feed.
- Inspect and palpate inside the mouth for cleft lip and palate, and check the sucking (or 'rooting') reflex (**Figure 2.4**).
- Check for a tongue tie if there are feeding concerns (**Figure 2.5**).
- Check for teeth. Congenital teeth are often loose and therefore pose a risk of aspiration or poor feeding. Refer these babies to a maxillofacial surgeon.
- Inspect for symmetry of facial movements: a common complication of forceps deliveries is a Bell's (facial nerve) palsy.

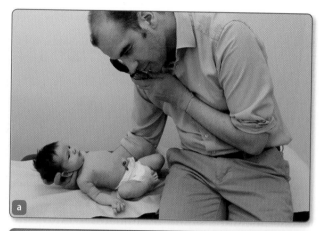

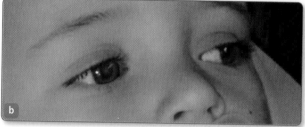

**Figure 2.3** (a) Elicit the red reflex by using an ophthalmoscope at a distance, rather than close up. (b) A normal red reflex is demonstrated in the right eye. The left eye shows worrying leucocoria.

## Skin

Of the many benign neonatal skin conditions, erythema toxicum is the most common. It presents as a small, raised white spot surrounded by a 1–2 mm ring of erythema. The spots may become confluent, resulting in a rash over all the trunk, but the baby is otherwise completely well (**Figure 2.6**).

Note the presence of birthmarks (see page 255).

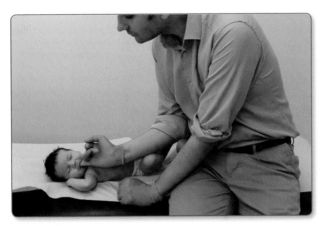

**Figure 2.4** The sucking reflex. If the cheek is rubbed, the baby turns the head to the side and searches for a nipple ('rooting'). They then suck strongly in a coordinated fashion.

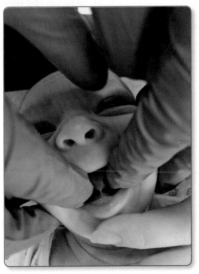

**Figure 2.5** Tongue-tie. The tip of the tongue is tethered by a fibrous band.

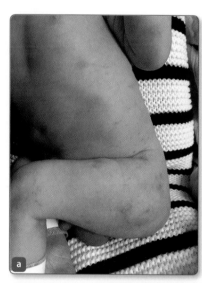

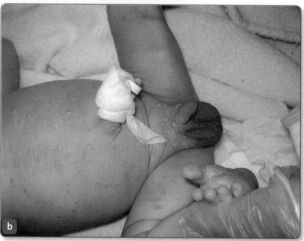

**Figure 2.6** (a) Erythema toxicum is a benign rash characterised by tense yellow spots with an erythematous halo. (b) The spots of benign pustular melanosis are flaccid but are not suggestive of infection – there is no erythema.

## Clavicles

The clavicle can be fractured during an obstructed labour. Palpate along the length of the bone for crepitus or swelling.

## Arms

Observe the arms for signs of brachial plexus injury:

- Erb's palsy (damage to superior nerve roots) – the affected arm is extended with the wrist flexed (the 'waiter's tip' posture)
- Klumpke's palsy (damage to the inferior nerve roots) – the arm is held flexed across the body (the 'Napoleon' posture)

## Hands

A single palmar crease may be seen in healthy babies but is a feature of Down's syndrome (see page 287).

Look at the shape and number of fingers, noting any that are fused (syndactyly), or small and curved (clinodactyly). Extra (accessory) digits may be small and tethered to the adjacent finger by a small skin bridge. Preaxial (radial/thumb side) are

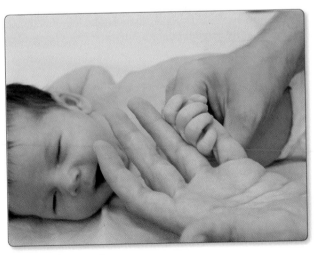

Figure 2.7 The grasp reflex.

often associated with other congenital abnormalities; postaxial (ulnar/little finger side) ones are often benign.

Check the grasp reflex (**Figure 2.7**). An absent grasp reflex may be a sign of nerve damage or brain injury.

## Chest

Abnormal chest shapes, such as pectus carinatum ('pigeon chest') and pectus excavatum (a deeply recessed sternum), can cause problems with respiration.

Count the respiratory rate and observe for signs of respiratory distress (see page 37). These can signify sepsis, hypoglycaemia, hypercarbia or hypoxia.

Hyperplasia of breast tissue and even lactation may be observed in neonates as a result of maternal prolactin crossing the placenta. This resolves spontaneously.

Auscultate for equal bilateral breath sounds. Pneumothorax is a common cause of deterioration in neonates.

## Heart

Listen to the heart sounds in all four areas (**Figure 2.8**). A crying baby may settle if sucking on a finger or given oral sucrose. Heart murmurs should be investigated using four-limb blood pressures and bilateral oxygen saturations (see **Chapter 7**).

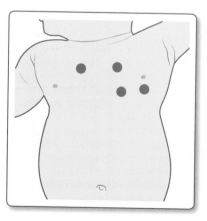

**Figure 2.8** Listening to the heart sounds. Place the stethoscope in all four auscultatory regions.

## Femoral pulses

The femoral pulse is located about halfway along the inguinal ligament, which runs between the symphysis pubis and iliac crest. An impalpable femoral pulse may indicate coarctation of the aorta and requires an urgent echocardiogram.

## Abdomen

Palpate for organomegaly (**Figure 2.9**). A 1 cm liver edge is normal.

An omphalocoele, in which the abdomen is open and the viscera are exposed, requires urgent surgery. However, an umbilical hernia is quite common and usually resolves spontaneously if managed conservatively.

The umbilical stump should be clean and dry. Infection from the umbilical stump (omphalitis) can spread rapidly to the liver, which may feel 'woody' and be very tender. Malodorous or red periumbilical skin should therefore be treated with intravenous antibiotics.

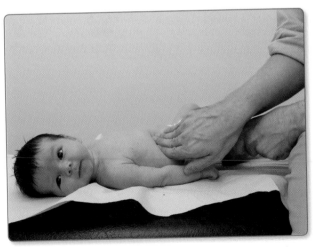

**Figure 2.9** Palpating the abdomen gently, with the radial border of the index finger, to feel for a liver edge that moves with respiration.

## Groin

If a hernia is present, refer the baby to a paediatric surgeon. An inguinal hernia in a girl may contain the ovary.

## Genitalia

### In boys

Inspect the penis for the urethral meatus, which may be sited on the dorsum (epispadias) or ventral shaft (hypospadias).

Palpate the testes to check they have descended. Retractile testes are located in the inguinal region but can easily be brought down. If a testis is impalpable, ultrasound and surgical referral are required.

### In girls

The genitalia may be virilised in conditions such as congenital adrenal hyperplasia. Falling levels of maternal progesterone can cause minor withdrawal bleeding from the baby's vagina.

### Clinical insight

When examining the spine and buttocks, blue spot birthmarks (**Figure 2.11**) must be clearly documented to prevent them subsequently being mistaken for bruises.

### Legs

Look for talipes equinovarus (club foot; **Figure 2.10**). If present, assess whether it is postural (the foot can be

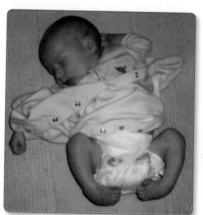

**Figure 2.10** Talipes equinovarus.

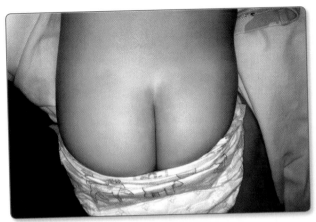

Figure 2.11 A blue spot birthmark can be confused with an extensive bruise.

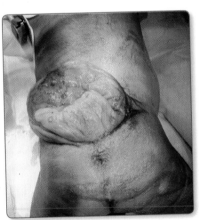

Figure 2.12 Spina bifida – herniation of the dura through an unfused spine. This baby has been washed with povidone-iodine antiseptic in preparation for surgery.

straightened) or fixed (the curved shape of the foot cannot be returned to normal by stretching).

## Spina bifida

True spina bifida (**Figure 2.12**) is rare in countries where folate is routinely given to women during the first trimester of pregnancy.

Look for tufts of hair or pits in the natal cleft. Pits in the natal cleft are common and only of concern if the base of the pit cannot be seen. In this case, ultrasound will ascertain whether the pit extends down to the spinal cord.

## Anus

Check for a visible anus. As meconium can be passed through a fistula or via the vagina, a history of opening the bowels is not enough to exclude low rectal or anal atresia. Imperforate anus is part of VACTERL syndrome (vertebral defects, anal atresia, cardiac defects, tracheo-oesophageal fistula, renal abnormalities and limb abnormalities) and requires urgent echocardiogram, renal ultrasound and surgical referral.

## Reflexes

Examination of the reflexes and hips is best left until the end of the neonatal examination, because the palpation and manipulation involved are likely to make the baby cry. If this happens, it impedes subsequent cardiac, abdominal and ocular examination.

### Moro reflex

Support the baby's back with one hand, and the head with the other (**Figure 2.13**). Quickly bring both hands down by approximately 2 or 3 cm so the baby momentarily falls backwards. The baby should throw both arms out symmetrically and then bring the forearms together towards the midline.

The Moro reflex may be asymmetrical in peripheral nerve damage, such as brachial plexus injury. An overpronounced or totally absent Moro reflex both indicate hypoxic–ischaemic encephalopathy.

### Stepping reflex

The stepping reflex (**Figure 2.14**) is elicited by holding the baby in a standing position and slowly moving them forwards with their toes touching the bed. The baby will lift the feet and place them in front of each other, as if walking.

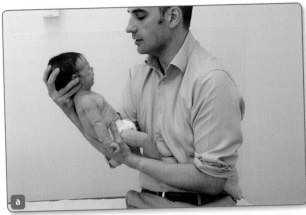

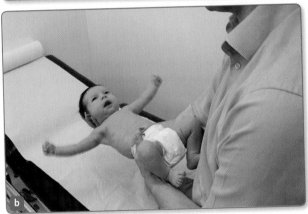

**Figure 2.13** Eliciting the Moro reflex. From the position shown, let the baby's head fall back gently by 2–3 cm. The baby will fling out the arms in a 'startle' or Moro reflex.

## Hips

The Barlow and Ortolani tests help to rule out developmental dysplasia of the hip, in which the acetabulum does not form properly. This condition can irreversibly limit motor development if not isolated and treated early. If the Barlow or Ortolani

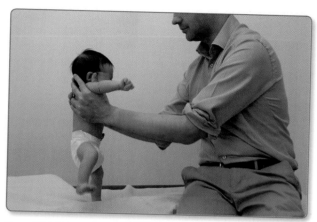

**Figure 2.14** The stepping reflex.

test is positive, (an audible clunk or click) then the femoral head is dislocatable from a malformed socket. A normal baby will have negative Barlow and Ortolani's tests.

### Barlow test

The Barlow test (**Figure 2.15**) examines whether the head of the femur can be dislocated posteriorly.

With the baby lying supine, bring the legs to the midline and flex the knees to 90°. With an index finger on the greater trochanter of each femur, push the knees down towards the bed. There may be a palpable 'clunk 'if the hip dislocates.

### Clinical insight

You can remember how each hip test is performed by remembering 'Barlow = back, Ortolani = open.'

### Ortolani test

The Ortolani test (**Figure 2.16**) aims to relocate a hip that is already dislocated. With the baby's knees flexed to 90° and touching each other,

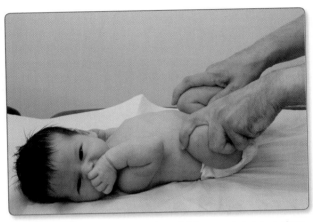

**Figure 2.15** The Barlow test. See if the hip will dislocate posteriorly by pushing the femur backwards, out of the acetabulum.

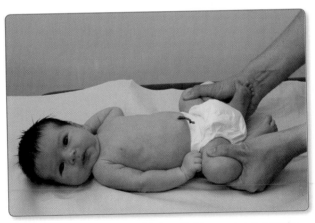

**Figure 2.16** The Ortolani test. See if the hip will dislocate anteriorly. Bring the head of the femur forwards out of the acetabulum by palpating the greater trochanter and opening out the hips.

place an index finger on the greater trochanter and externally rotate the femurs, opening up the legs. There will be a 'click' if the head of a dislocated femur pops back into the acetabulum.

## 2.5 Examination summary

The newborn examination is summarised in **Table 2.5**.

| Component | Key findings |
|---|---|
| Colour | Jaundice, plethora, cyanosis, petechiae, mottling |
| Head | Dysmorphia, cranial sutures, cleft palate, suck, ear abnormalities, red reflex |
| Limbs | Number of palmar creases, polydactyly, syndactyly, talipes, palsies, hip dislocation |
| Chest | Clavicular fractures, chest shape, breath and heart sounds |
| Abdomen | Organomegaly, hernias, umbilical cord |
| Back | Spinal pits, blue spot, muscle tone, anus |
| Genitalia | Position of testes, abnormal genitalia |
| Reflexes | Moro, stepping |
| Have you ruled out … ? | Sepsis, genetic syndrome, heart failure, respiratory distress |

**Table 2.5** Summary of the newborn examination

# The child

Whereas there is a single systematic approach for examining a newborn, this is not true for most children. Most consultations are for an acute or chronic health problem, not for routine screening. Furthermore, they do not necessarily cooperate with an examination. They are often unwell, irascible and scared, and they also require a more focused examination relating to the presenting problem.

Each subsequent chapter focuses on the examination of a particular organ system (e.g. respiratory – see **Chapter 6**) or an area unique to paediatrics (e.g. growth – see **Chapter 4**). This chapter covers overarching principles that can be employed regardless of the focus of the clinical encounter.

Examination of children poses many challenges:

- Children often do not want to be examined
- Young children, even if compliant, struggle to follow complex instructions
- A child's size and fat distribution frequently make simple assessments, e.g. pulse taking, challenging
- Their health can improve and deteriorate quickly
- There is often a mismatch between the severity of the reported symptoms and the clinical assessment
- They require different approaches tailored to their age
- Non-verbal children cannot articulate subjective symptoms, e.g. pain
- Their physiology changes with age (**Table 3.1**)
- They have anatomical features such as fontanelles and a thymus that disappear over time
- They are not little adults (see **Chapter 1**)

## Clinical insight

Examination begins before you call the patient. Watch the child playing in the waiting area. A happy child who is playing but using only one hand may have a pulled elbow. A 5-year-old who is sitting quietly and not interacting may be very sick.

| Age | Pulse (beats per minute) | Systolic blood pressure (mmHg) | Respiratory rate (breaths per minute) |
|---|---|---|---|
| 0–3 months | 100–160 | 70–90 | 30–60 |
| 3–12 months | 100–160 | 70–90 | 30–50 |
| 1–5 years | 90–140 | 80–100 | 22–40 |
| 5–12 years | 80–120 | 90–110 | 20–25 |
| >12 years | 60–100 | 100–120 | 12–20 |

**Table 3.1** Pulse, systolic blood pressure and respiratory rate: normal values according to age

# 3.1 Recognising the sick child

It may be difficult to recognise when children are sick, especially if you are new to working with them. Children have different physiological normal values from adults (see **Table 3.1**), and these parameters also have a different sensitivity and specificity for disease severity .

Unlike adults, children maintain their blood pressure in the early phases of serious illness. Hypotension is a very late sign in childhood diseases, and a rising heart rate is a much more sensitive physiological indicator of disease progression. An active, screaming child usually has a good clinical prognosis; a quiet, subdued child is more worrying as they can be in significant pain or lethargic.

## Clinical insight

In children <5 years of age, the severity of an infection cannot be assessed by the height of a fever. A child with a temperature of 38°C may be septic, whereas a child with a temperature of 41°C may just have a middle ear infection

## Red flags

As well as 'red flag' symptoms identified in the clinical history (see **Chapter 1**), red flag signs are elicited during observation and examination. Respiratory distress is the most common red flag sign in acute medicine. Online videos will help you familiarize yourself with these unusual breathing patterns.

Red flag signs in the examination include:

- lethargy and poor interaction
- fever over 38°C in an unvaccinated or partially vaccinated baby
- respiratory distress (**Table 3.2**)
- a non-blanching rash
- green vomit
- cool peripheries
- prolonged capillary refill
- decreased consciousness
- anuria
- haemorrhage
- abnormal respiratory rate
- abnormal heart rate
- hypotension

## Clinical insight

A baby <4 months old with a fever >38°C must be treated with intravenous antibiotics and be given a diagnosis of possible sepsis until proven otherwise. A full septic screen should be performed, including chest radiograph, urine culture, blood culture and lumbar puncture.

## 3.2 Recognising the abused child

Safeguarding is a priority when examining a child. Abuse usually falls into one or more of four categories: physical, psychological, sexual and neglect. As well as red flags in the history (see **Chapter 1**), signs on examination should prompt discussion with a senior colleague. These include:

- an unkempt in child in dirty, smelly, ill-fitting clothes

| Distress | Description |
|---|---|
| Nasal flare | Nostrils widen during inspiration |
| Tracheal tug | Throat dips during inspiration (caused by downward traction of bronchial tree) |
| Recession | Part of chest wall draws in during inspiration  May be subcostal, intercostal or sternal |
| Grunting | Airway briefly occludes at the larynx during expiration in an attempt to maintain a positive end expiratory pressure |
| See-saw breathing | Chest moves inwards and abdomen outwards during inspiration; the reverse occurs in expiration |

**Table 3.2** Types of respiratory distress

- visible malnourishment
- abnormal interaction with the parent
- bruising over non-bony areas, e.g. the buttocks
- multiple scars or blemishes
- comprehension of sexual behaviour that is abnormal for the child's age
- bruising to the genitalia or anus
- an injury incompatible with the history given

## 3.3 Examination of a child

There should ideally be:
- a warm and clean environment
- toys and games available
- a stethoscope, otoscope and tongue depressor
- someone to help – a nurse or play specialist
- patience and flexibility

### Environment and equipment

Aim to create an environment in which a child feels safe (**Figure 3.1**). Toys, books, portable DVD players and tablet

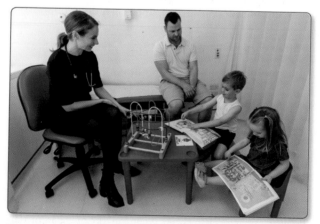

**Figure 3.1** A child-friendly environment for clinical examinations.

computers are routine equipment to have available. Consider the micro- and macroenvironment; for example, examine younger children on their parent's lap while they are cuddling their favourite blanket, in a warm room so that the child is comfortable when undressed.

Procedures that are frightening or uncomfortable, such as blood taking, should ideally be done in a separate room specifically designed for this purpose. Useful equipment is then easily to hand, and this also allows children to consider the bed space or waiting room as a 'safe space'.

It is not appropriate to offer edible rewards such as sweets, because many children you see will have allergies, diabetes or metabolic disease, or are not tolerating an oral intake. Instead, a clinic should have a supply of other treats, such as stickers.

## Nurses and play specialists

Nursing staff can help distract children during examination and also act as chaperones when older children are being examined by a clinician. Play specialists use play therapy to distract and comfort children of all ages during painful procedures such as cannulation. Useful distraction techniques include:

- blowing bubbles
- following a story or describing a picture
- watching a video on a tablet or smartphone
- playing 'I spy'
- getting older children to recount a story

## Flexibility: performance and language

You do not need to use a rigid series of steps when examining children. There is no need always to start with their hands; instead, start with the important or practical, and work from there. If the child is shy and clingy, start with the areas that the parents can help show you, such as exposing the chest to look for respiratory distress.

Try to examine children in an age-appropriate way, which is often best done through mimicry. Get down to their level, mentally and physically – on the knees if examining small children – or even below them while they are on a parent's lap

(**Figure 3.2**). Looming over young children scares them. Parents and toys are a useful resource – examine the parent or teddy bear first to reassure the child.

Use age-appropriate language and try to avoid jargon. A 5-year-old will not understand 'abdomen' or 'spine' but will understand 'tummy' and 'back'. Do not be too self-conscious – young children enjoy silly humour and funny noises, and turning a clinical examination into a game is a good way to win them over. With adolescents, adopt an attitude that is suitable for a young adult; practitioners who patronise adolescents are unlikely to build good therapeutic relationships with them.

## Clinical insight

Avoid urging young children to be 'brave'. Children know that bravery is needed when something painful or unpleasant is going to happen. You are inadvertently suggesting that your examination is going to hurt.

### Parents

Parents are your greatest allies in helping to examine the child. They can dress and undress toddlers without scaring them, and provide soothing cuddles and reassurance. They are also

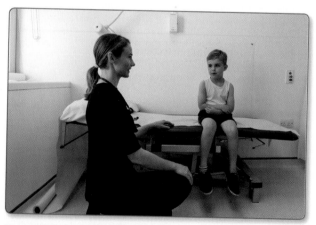

**Figure 3.2** Getting down to the child's level.

best placed to hold their child for some of the more uncomfortable examinations, such as ear and throat examinations (see **Chapter 11**).

## Cultural considerations

Patients from different cultural backgrounds often have different expectations about the practitioner–patient relationship. Be aware that some examinations that do not feel intimate to you can be perceived as intimate to a patient or their family. This could include examining the scalp of a child who usually wears religious head-coverings, or examining a rash on a patient's shins.

Do not behave as if everything is routine. Ask both the child and parent about their ideas, concerns and expectations. This is especially important if a genital examination is required.

> ### Clinical insight
>
> Examine as much of the child as possible, within reason. Many paediatric conditions present with rashes, which are easily missed if a healthcare practitioner is worried about exposing the child.

## Crying and tantrums

### Examining the crying baby

Persistent crying is a sign in itself. Is it due to irritability? Tiredness? Hunger? The need for a nappy change? A baby should settle when comforted by a parent, or with a dummy or a feed. This provides an opportunity to listen to the heart and breath sounds. If the parents are not present, a nurse can console the baby, or the baby can be given a sucrose solution. If the baby remains unhappy, consider that this may be a sign of illness and ask a more senior clinician.

### Examining the unhappy toddler

If a toddler (a 1- to 3-year-old) is upset and unwilling to be examined, try another approach. Encourage the child's attention by pretending to examine their teddy bear or a sibling; the child often then demands their 'turn'. A firm chest-to-chest hug from the parent allows access so that the back can be auscultated and the abdomen palpated. The stethoscope can then be worked

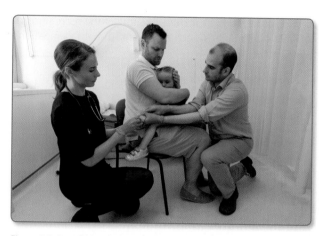

**Figure 3.3** An unhappy toddler can be examined or cannulated when chest-to-chest with a parent. The parent can steady the child's arms under their own to prevent flailing. A colleague or second parent can provide playful distraction or a steadying hand.

round to the front to auscultate the heart sounds. This is also a good position to examine for cervical lymphadenopathy and take blood (**Figure 3.3**).

## 3.4 Chaperones

Do not place yourself at risk when performing intimate examinations of a child. You should not perform an examination of the genitalia in a child of any age, or of the breasts when they have developed, unless a chaperone is present. The presence of a parent is not adequate. Chaperones are particularly important if an older child asks to be examined without their parent in the room, for example when looking for evidence of self-harm.

It is best, but not essential, for the chaperone to be the same gender as the patient. Nurses and play therapists are ideally qualified to act as chaperones.

| Principle | Examples |
|---|---|
| Environment | Clean, colourful toys and games |
| Language | Age appropriate, jargon free |
| Distraction | Parent, colleague, bubbles, games, videos |
| Approach | Patient height, non threatening, chaperones, examine relative or toy |
| Have you ruled out … ? | Severe illness, child abuse |

Table 3.3 Summary of paediatric examination principles

## 3.5 Examination summary

The guiding principles of paediatric examination are shown in **Table 3.3**.

## chapter 4

# Growth and nutrition

Children vary in their diet and metabolic needs more than any other patient population. Unlike adults, children need to ingest extra calories on top of their basic metabolic requirement in order to grow and develop. In assessing growth, there is a focus on height, weight and head measurements because aberrations can be significant warning signs of disease or worrying social circumstances.

The rate of growth varies throughout life, being highest during infancy and puberty. Greatest growth occurs during the first year: children usually triple their birth weight by 12 months of age. Their calorie requirement in the first year is three times that of an adult (approximately 100 kcal/kg per day – which equates to approximately 150 mL/kg per day of milk). Breast milk has advantages over formula milk (**Table 4.1**), unless contraindicated (**Table 4.2**). Premature babies, with higher heart and respiratory

| Property | Benefit |
|---|---|
| Immunity | Maternal IgA transfers to the baby |
| Digestion | Human long-chain fatty acid molecules are easier to digest |
| Reduced risk of severe disease | Reduced risk of SIDS and leukaemia |
| Long-term health | Correlates with reduced risk of obesity and diabetes |
| Reduced risk of allergies | Less allergenic itself, and correlates with reduced incidence of allergies in children with a family history of atopy |
| Maternal health | Reduces risk of breast and ovarian cancer, diabetes and heart disease |
| SIDS, sudden infant death syndrome. | |

**Table 4.1** Benefits of breastfeeding over formula milk

| Category | Examples |
|---|---|
| Metabolic | Galactosaemia, lactose intolerance |
| Medication | Lithium, benzodiazepines, ergots |
| Illicit drug use | Opiates, benzodiazepines, alcohol |
| Malignancy | Chemotherapy, radiotherapy |
| Radioisotopes | Iodine-131, technetium-99 m |
| Systemic infection | Tuberculosis, varicella zoster virus, HIV* |
| Local infection | Mastitis, herpetic lesions |

*In developed countries maternal HIV is a contraindication. However, in countries where water supplies are not clean, risk of water-borne infections may be greater than risk of vertical transmission of HIV.

Table 4.2  Contraindications to breastfeeding

rates, have an even higher calorie demand, requiring 180 mL/kg or even 200 mL/kg per day of milk for growth.

## Presentation of poor growth

When infants wean onto solid foods at 4–6 months of age, oral fluid requirements fall substantially, but the variety of digestive processes required to metabolise the increased variety food increases. This creates a specific window between 4 and 9 months of age when previously dormant pathologies relating to allergy, intolerance or metabolic dysfunction are able to manifest.

In childhood, poor growth is a common presentation. Older children are often conscious of their height and weight in comparison to their peers, and can be distressed when they feel that they are not physically developing in the same way as their friends.

### Clinical insight

A contraindication to breastfeeding does not necessarily mean that breast milk is contraindicated. Children with a cleft palate, for example, can take breast milk from specially adapted bottles. Babies whose mothers are receiving cytotoxic medications can have breast milk from a donor.

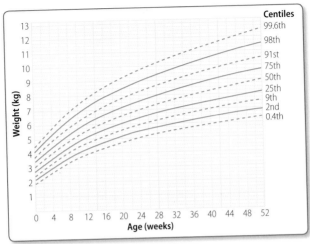

**Figure 4.1** A standard World Health Organization paediatric growth chart for a girl aged 1 year.

Poor growth is also a common chance discovery on examination. Therefore, each of the following chapters on the organ systems in paediatric examination repeats the need to record the child's height and weight on a growth chart (**Figure 4.1**).

## 4.1 Clinical scenarios

### Poor weight gain

An 18-month-old boy who was born in a country that does not have newborn screening is referred to the paediatric clinic because his parents are concerned about his weight. He had a normal birthweight (3.7 kg, 75th centile) but at 1 year of age he weighed 8.2 kg (9th centile) and now weighs 8.6 kg (2nd centile).

### Differential diagnosis

The child has failure to thrive. The following possibilities should be considered:
- inadequate nutritional intake

- malabsorption
- increased losses
- increased use of calories

## Further information

There is no history of poor feeding and he appears cared for. His bowel habit is unusual, producing bulky, explosive, porridge-like stools three to four times a day. He had seven lower respiratory infections in his first year of life; these required antibiotics due to prolonged symptoms that were slow to resolve.

## Conclusion

The repeated lower respiratory tract infections suggest that this child has an underlying immunodeficiency syndrome. It is unusual to have seven bacterial chest infections in a year. He should have a full blood count (FBC), immunoglobulins and vaccine responses tested. Second line tests include a sweat test for cystic fibrosis, along with lymphocyte subsets and a neutrophil burst test. A referral to immunology is required if the sweat test is normal. In this case, cystic fibrosis is most likely, as it also explains the diarrhoea.

## Shortest boy in the class

A boy aged 14 years and 6 months presents to the clinic, very self-conscious that he is lagging behind his peers in terms of growth and development. He was of average height for his class up to the age of 11 but is now the shortest. He is being teased at school for 'being short and having a high-pitched voice'. His current height is 155 cm.

## Differential diagnosis

Potential causes of reduced growth velocity are:

- nutritional deficiency
- malabsorption
- neglect
- increased metabolic demands
- constitutional pubertal delay
- growth hormone/gonadotropin deficiency

## Further information

The boy was born after an unremarkable pregnancy with growth on the 50th centile. His father is 177 cm tall, and his mother 163 cm. Approximately a year ago, he was seen in the emergency department for a soft tissue injury; his height was then recorded as 150 cm. He has a balanced diet and is excelling academically. Bowel habit is normal, and there are no recurrent infections. On examination, the testes are 8 mL in volume, and there is scant pubic hair and a small amount of hair in the left axilla. A radiograph of the wrist shows a bone age of 13 years.

## Conclusion

This is constitutional pubertal delay. He is at Tanner stage 2–3 of puberty (see pages 61–63) with a growth velocity of 5 cm/year, which will increase to 8 cm/year as he progresses through puberty. The mid-parental height is 177 cm, which the boy will probably achieve by 19–20 years of age.

# 4.2 Common presentations

Growth problems classically present as:
- neonatal weight loss
- faltering weight
- abnormal growth pattern

## Neonatal weight loss

Babies can lose up to 10% of their body weight in the first 5 days of life, as water, meconium and fat are lost. With time, as milk intake increases, growth starts in earnest. Babies are expected re-achieve their birthweight within the first 2 weeks of life.

A loss of >10% of body weight or a failure to regain birthweight in 3 weeks can be caused by:
- feeding difficulties
- milk allergy or lactose intolerance

### Clinical insight

Approximately 10% of the protein in breast milk is maternal immunoglobulin (IgA), which provides immune protection to the newborn as its own immune system develops.

- congenital disorders
- malabsorption
- infection

## Primary lactation difficulties

Lactation is not as easy as many parents presume: it is commonly delayed in women who have traumatic or caesarean deliveries, and can be difficult to establish or be interrupted by illness or mastitis. It is also very difficult to judge how much milk a baby is ingesting: a baby will fall asleep after 20 minutes on a full breast through satiety, or on an empty breast through exhaustion.

> ## Clinical insight
>
> Medical professionals often use the word 'failure' to describe an unsuccessful process, as in 'growth failure' and 'lactation failure'. This can feel judgemental to parents so avoid it and instead use 'difficulties' or 'problem'.

*Clinical features*  The baby may be thin with loose skin folds, a sunken anterior fontanelle and a dry mouth. In severe cases, the baby becomes sleepy and jaundiced. Hypernatraemic dehydration and hypoglycaemia are potentially dangerous situations because there is a risk of a stroke or seizures.

## Milk allergy or lactose intolerance

Cow's milk allergy is not limited to bottle-fed infants: maternally-ingested cow's milk protein is absorbed into breast milk.

*Clinical features*  Constipation or, more commonly, diarrhoea, is characteristic, particularly in lactose intolerance. Here the stool is foul-smelling and acidic, leading to marked perianal excoriation. Other symptoms include abdominal pain, vomiting, discomfort on feeding, and blood in the stool.

## Congenital causes

The numerous congenital causes of poor weight gain in the neonatal period are physical or metabolic.

**Physical barriers to feeding**  The clinical assessment must exclude all of the many physical problems affecting feeding. Key causes include:

- cleft palate
- tongue-tie
- abnormalities of the chin (e.g. micrognathia in Pierre Robin sequence)
- choanal atresia, in which the nasal passages are not patent, so the infant cannot breathe when feeding

**Increased metabolic demand**  Any condition producing a higher need for calories leads to poor growth. Common causes include:

- chronic respiratory illness with tachypnoea (e.g. chronic lung disease of prematurity)
- congenital cardiac disease (see **Chapter 7**)
- infection, e.g. urinary tract infection (see page 126)
- chronic or multiple infections, e.g. HIV and severe combined immunodeficiency (SCID)
- inborn errors of metabolism – many rare disorders involve enzyme deficiencies

## Faltering weight

Faltering weight is usually defined as the crossing of 2 centiles on the growth chart. If the weight was below the 2nd centile at birth, crossing 1 centile is sufficient to define faltering growth.

The causes can be broadly divided into:

- lack of intake
- vitamin deficiency
- excess losses (from vomiting, diarrhoea or malabsorption)
- increased metabolic demand (see above)

### Lack of intake

Inadequate calorie intake can result from:

- inadequate offered milk, e.g. lactation failure
- weaning failure
- behavioural feeding problems

> ## Clinical insight
>
> Iron deficiency is a common result of failure to wean. This results in severe anaemia, with haemoglobin levels as low as 30 g/L (normal 110–140 g/L). Iron deficiency causes abnormalities in appetite and gustation, regardless of anaemia. Treating it may help to reduce dietary fussiness.

**Inadequate milk offered**  Inadequate milk is caused by lactation difficulties, as outlined above, or the infant requiring more milk than is being offered. Inadequate offering of milk is either innocent or deliberate, but requires urgent intervention and escalation whatever the cause.

**Weaning failure**  Most infants are weaned on to solids by 6 months of age and drink progressively less milk as the solid diet becomes more established. Both the quality and quantity of breast milk tend to lessen beyond 6 months, and may not subsequently be adequate to meet the infant's total needs. Infants who fail to start weaning around this age are at significant risk of insufficient calorie intake and micronutrient deficiencies.

**Behavioural feeding problems**  A reluctance or refusal to ingest milk or solids is common. It often follows on from an earlier period when feeding was associated with pain, for example with reflux or allergy. In severe cases, this requires temporary nasogastric feeding and the support of a feeding team including speech and language therapists and psychologists.

Eating disorders are increasingly common in teenagers, particularly girls. These conditions are dealt with in more detail in **Chapter 13**.

## Clinical insight

Fat-soluble vitamins are particularly susceptible to malabsorption, for example in pancreatic insufficiency caused by cystic fibrosis. The fat-soluble nutrients can be remembered from the mnemonic **DALEK**, where each letter stands for a vitamin, apart from L, which stands for 'lipids'.

### Vitamin and iron deficiencies

Adequate quantities of vitamins and minerals are needed for normal growth. The most common deficiencies are shown in **Table 4.3**.

### Excess losses

Losses may be obvious (e.g. from vomiting or frank diarrhoea – see **Chapter 8**) or less obvious (e.g. from malabsorption, in which the stools can be simply bulky and smelly – see **Chapter 8**).

Common causes of excess losses include:
- gastro-oesophageal reflux (see page 130)
- pyloric stenosis (see page 131)

| Deficiency | Symptoms | Causes |
|---|---|---|
| Vitamin D | Lethargy, bone pain, leg bowing, cardiomyopathy | Poor exposure to sunlight, pancreatic insufficiency, late weaning |
| Iron | Anaemia, lethargy, fussy eating | Vegetarianism, heavy periods, late weaning |
| Vitamin K | Increased risk of bleeding | Pancreatic insufficiency, lack of administration at birth |
| Zinc | Facial and groin skin breakdown | Acrodermatitis enteropathica |
| Vitamin C | Mucosal and skin ulceration, tooth loss, poor skin healing | – |
| Vitamin E | Neurological deterioration | Pancreatic insufficiency |
| Vitamin A | Reduced visual acuity | Pancreatic insufficiency |

Table 4.3 Common vitamin and mineral deficiencies

- lactose intolerance (see page 50)
- cystic fibrosis
- coeliac disease (see page 133)
- inflammatory bowel disease (see page 128)
- inborn errors of metabolism
- malignancy

## Abnormal growth

The five main presentations of abnormal growth are:
- disproportionate head circumference
- short stature
- pubertal delay
- abnormal growth acceleration
- precocious puberty

## Disproportionate head circumference

**Table 4.4** details the common causes of abnormal head circumference. A head measuring below the 0.4th centile is classed as microcephalic, and one above the 99.6th centile as macrocephalic. These are occasionally normal findings,

| Microcephaly | Macrocephaly |
|---|---|
| • Genetic syndromes, e.g. Down's syndrome<br>• Prenatal infection, e.g. cytomegalovirus, Zika virus<br>• Prenatal ischaemia<br>• Prenatal toxin, e.g. fetal alcohol syndrome<br>• Craniosynostosis (premature fusion of the sutures) | • Familial<br>• Fragile X syndrome<br>• Overgrowth conditions, e.g. Sotos syndrome<br>• Hydrocephalus<br>• Trauma, e.g. subgaleal collection |

**Table 4.4** Causes of abnormal head circumference

particularly when in proportion to the rest of the child, but they always merit investigation.

### Abnormal stature

The main causes of abnormal stature to consider are:
• familial stature
• constitutional delay of growth
• growth hormone abnormalities
• genetic syndromes
• pubertal dysregulation
• chronic illness, including malnutrition

**Familial stature** A child with familial causes of abnormal stature falls within the expected centile range, based on the mid-parental height (see below). The growth velocity measured over a minimum of 6 months is normal.

**Clinical insight**

A good indicator of whether growth is stopping or likely to continue is fusion of the growth plates. A wrist radiograph can therefore reassure children with constitutionally delayed puberty that they have 'a lot of growing left in them'. These children have a bone age a year or so lower than their chronological age.

**Constitutional delay of growth** A child with constitutional growth delay has no underlying abnormality, and although the child may appear to be falling off the normal growth centiles, they eventually catch up once puberty commences.

**Growth hormone abnormalities**  Growth hormone excess or deficiency is:
- idiopathic
- secondary to pituitary dysfunction, e.g. with a pituitary tumour or following irradiation

In a child with growth hormone deficiency, growth velocity falls below the minimum (4 cm/year) that is required for normal growth. The child can also appear slightly overweight. A child with an excess of growth hormone has a growth velocity well above normal and may develop acromegalic features.

**Genetic syndromes**  Many syndromes are associated with short stature (see also **Chapter 14**). They include:
- achondroplasia
- hypochondroplasia
- Down's syndrome
- Turner's syndrome
- Noonan's syndrome
- Prader–Willi syndrome
- Silver–Russell syndrome
- *SHOX* homeobox mutations

Abnormally tall stature has fewer genetic differential diagnoses. The most common is Marfan's syndrome (see page 296).

**Pubertal dysregulation**  The growth spurt occurs during puberty. Children who go through puberty later than their peers are significantly shorter than their friends during adolescence. However, they catch up as their classmates' growth spurts come to an end.

More concerning are children who start puberty early. Early puberty signals the growth plates to fuse and growth to stop far earlier than normal. Precocious puberty causes a child to be initially tall in their class, but in the long term is a cause of significant short stature.

## Clinical insight

Any poorly controlled chronic illness can cause growth delay. Furthermore, the treatment of some chronic diseases involves regular corticosteroids; even if only inhaled, these can cause a reduction in growth velocity.

## 4.3 Examination of growth

The examination of a child's growth comprises:
- general inspection
- formal auxology
- systems review
- pubertal assessment
- further investigations

### General inspection

Look for:
- dysmorphic features (see **Chapter 14**)
- loose skin folds (malnutrition)
- abdominal distension (malabsorption – see page 133)
- rapport with the parent or carer
- signs of neglect
- bowed legs (rickets)

### Auxology

Auxology is the measurement of:
- height (or length in a baby) (**Figure 4.2**)
- arm span
- head circumference (**Figure 4.3**)
- weight
- growth velocity
- growth targets

These measurements should be plotted on an appropriate growth chart and adjusted for prematurity (**Figure 4.4**). Plotting a child on the wrong chart will yield incorrect centiles and cause unnecessary concerns about their growth velocity (Figure 4.5). Separate growth charts are available for:
- different sexes
- different age ranges
- specific conditions (e.g. Down's syndrome – see **Figure 4.5** – and achondroplasia)

### Height

Height or length should be measured with the child's footwear removed. Ensure the child's posture maximises the height (see **Figure 4.2**).

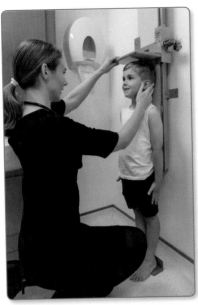

**Figure 4.2** Measure height with the child standing barefoot. Ensure the back is against the wall and the head straight.

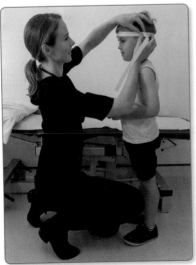

**Figure 4.3** Measurement of head circumference, horizontally around widest part of the occiput and forehead.

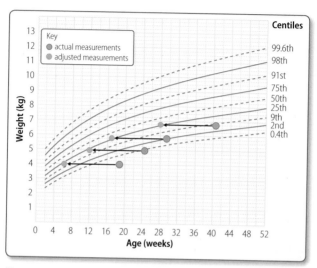

**Figure 4.4** For this girl born at 28 weeks' gestation, auxology is adjusted back, from right to left, by 12 weeks. Although the raw data (blue) look like she is crossing centiles, the adjusted data (green) show that she is following the 25th centile.

## Arm span

With children who are unable to stand or who have spinal deformities, height can be estimated by arm span. Arm-span is roughly equal to height, often marginally shorter.

An arm-span-to-height ratio >1.05 is a positive sign of Marfan's syndrome (see page 296).

## Head circumference

Wrap a tape measure around the occiput and the forehead as horizontally as possible to obtain the occipitofrontal circumference (see **Figure 4.3**). Microcephaly (<0.4th centile) and macrocephaly (>99.6th centile) require investigation.

## Weight

Weight should be measured with the child as naked as possible. For babies, this means without a nappy. Older children should ideally be weighed in their underwear, and their shoes should be removed.

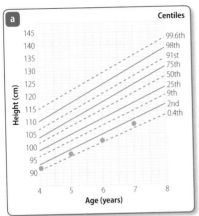

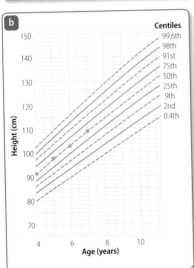

**Figure 4.5** Height for a child with Down's syndrome plotted on (a) a normal growth chart (0.4th centile) (b) a Down's syndrome growth chart (50th centile).

Shy or distressed children may not comply with being weighed. The easiest solution is to weigh the child in the arms of their parent, then weigh the parent on their own and calculate the difference.

### Growth velocity

Growth velocity is measured in centimetres per year, and requires serial measurements to calculate it. It is usually calculated in clinic by doubling the child's increase in height over 6 months. Measurements should be plotted on a growth velocity chart (**Figure 4.6**), as velocity alters significantly with age.

### Growth targets

Growth targets are measurements that children are expected to achieve over time. These include:

- centiles
- body mass index (BMI)
- mid-parental height

**Centiles**  Height, weight and head circumference should be lie on similar centiles and maintain these centiles throughout life (no more than 2 centile lines deviation in each case).

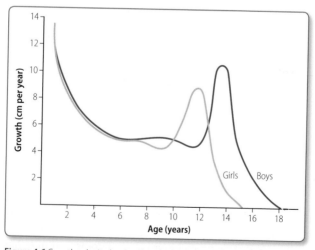

**Figure 4.6** Growth velocity (cm/year) comparing girls and boys. Note the 'growth spurt' at puberty.

Asymmetrical centiles (e.g. head growth on the 91st, but weight on the 9th, centile) warrant further investigation, as does a child who is 'crossing centiles'.

**BMI**  BMI targets in children alter with age. To calculate the BMI, divide the child's weight in kilograms by the square of their height in metres. The result should be plotted on an age-appropriate BMI chart, to calculate the BMI centile.

**Mid-parental height**  This is an estimation of a child's final adult height, and can be plotted at age 18 as a judge of what centile the child should be growing along. It is calculated by taking the mean average height of the child's biological parents and adjusting according to the sex of the child – adding 6.5 cm for a boy and deducting 6.5 cm for a girl.

## Systems review

Perform a general examination, which encapsulates most organ systems, looking for signs of chronic pathologies:
- hands for clubbing (see pages 96, 117)
- neck and axillae for lymphadenopathy (see page 224)
- sclerae for jaundice
- mouth for aphthous ulcers, e.g. in Crohn's disease (see page 128)
- conjunctivae for anaemia
- chest for heart murmurs (see page 107), crackles (see page 99) and 'rickety rosary' (a string-of-beads-like set of bumps where the ribs meet the sternum, caused by rickets)
- limbs for swelling and bowing
- abdomen for hepatosplenomegaly (see page 135)

## Pubertal status

Pubertal status should be examined when there is concern about growth in an older child. This involves examination of the genitalia (and in girls the chest as well). This should always be done with a chaperone present. Compare the physical findings with Tanner stages (**Figures 4.7** and **4.8**). When examining boys, palpate the testes and use an orchidometer (**Figure 4.9**) to judge their size.

The onset of menarche in girls and the development of facial hair in boys are secondary sexual characteristics and not part of the formal staging of puberty.

## Further investigations

Further investigations depend on clinical findings, but include:

- wrist radiography (for rickets or bone age – see page 54)
- MRI of the brain and pituitary
- blood tests, including thyroid function and pituitary and sex hormones
- karyotype (for Turner's or Down's syndrome)

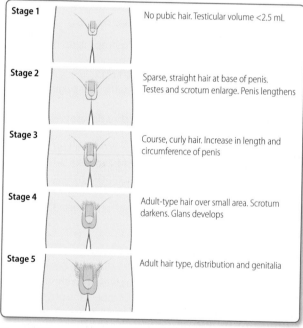

| Stage 1 | No pubic hair. Testicular volume <2.5 mL |
| Stage 2 | Sparse, straight hair at base of penis. Testes and scrotum enlarge. Penis lengthens |
| Stage 3 | Course, curly hair. Increase in length and circumference of penis |
| Stage 4 | Adult-type hair over small area. Scrotum darkens. Glans develops |
| Stage 5 | Adult hair type, distribution and genitalia |

**Figure 4.7** Tanner stages: male.

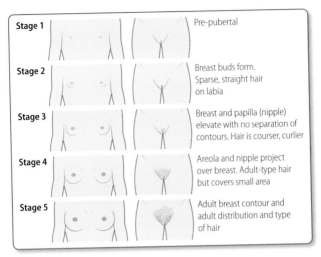

| Stage 1 | | | Pre-pubertal |
| Stage 2 | | | Breast buds form. Sparse, straight hair on labia |
| Stage 3 | | | Breast and papilla (nipple) elevate with no separation of contours. Hair is courser, curlier |
| Stage 4 | | | Areola and nipple project over breast. Adult-type hair but covers small area |
| Stage 5 | | | Adult breast contour and adult distribution and type of hair |

**Figure 4.8** Tanner stages: female.

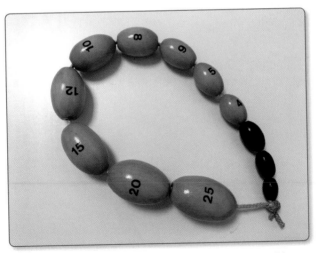

**Figure 4.9** An orchidometer. Each bead is labelled with its volume in millilitres.

## 4.4 Examination summary

A summary of the growth examination is given in **Table 4.5**.

| Component | Key findings |
|---|---|
| General inspection | Dysmorphia, abdominal distension, signs of neglect |
| Measurement | Height, weight, head circumference, arm span |
| Calculation | Adjustment for prematurity, growth velocity, mid-parental height, body mass index |
| Systems review | Clubbing, anaemia, lymphadenopathy, heart murmur, hepatosplenomegaly, leg bowing |
| Pubertal assessment | Tanner staging, secondary sexual characteristics |
| Investigations | Wrist radiography, karyotyping, thyroid function, specialist blood tests |
| Have you ruled out … ? | Neglect, failure to thrive, genetic syndromes, pubertal abnormalities, brain tumour |

**Table 4.5** Summary of growth examination and associated investigations

# Assessment of development

## chapter 5

Development is the sequential acquisition of new skills over the first few years of life. It should not be confused with growth or pubertal development (see **Chapter 4**), which is a physiological process. Development depends on four overlapping factors:

- the ability of sensory information to reach the brain
- the ability of the brain to process that information
- the opportunity of the child to practise skills
- the ability of the brain and motor structures to produce appropriate outputs

Development is classically broken down into four broad domains:

- gross and fine motor skills
- speech and language skills
- social skills and activities of daily living
- cognition and academic performance

Development occurs sequentially. There is a direct relationship between the development of gross motor skills (the intended movement of large muscle groups) and the length of the motor neurones. Hence full coordination of facial muscles occurs by 2 months of age. This is long before a baby is able to sit, for example, by 8 months, which requires trunk stability achieved by much longer neurones.

Many skills depend on previously acquired ones. For example, the use of cutlery – a 'social and personal' skill – depends on the timely acquisition of fine motor skills.

## 5.1 Clinical scenarios

Developmental delay can present in a single domain, or as global delay across multiple domains.

### A girl who is not sitting

A 10-month-old girl is referred by the health visitor. She is the first child of a single mother and was born at 39 weeks' gestation following a normal pregnancy. Antenatal scans and blood tests (including screening for Down's syndrome) were normal.

## Differential diagnosis

This includes:

- constitutional delay
- cerebral palsy
- spinal muscular atrophy
- muscular dystrophy
- Down's syndrome (see page 287)
- Prader–Willi syndrome (see page 294)
- hypothyroidism
- Rickets
- Neglect

## Further information

On examination, the child is propped up in a car seat. She is not dysmorphic but looks scrawny and is dressed in a dirty babygrow. She is not reaching out for objects but sits and cries until she is given a dummy or a bottle. She will turn to a sound and follow an object but does not interact with either.

Her mother is quiet and withdrawn, and smells of smoke. On discussing play, the mother bursts into tears and says she cannot play with her child but just places her in the car seat in front of the television.

## Conclusion

The girl is being neglected: her mother is suffering from depression and is struggling to cope. As the child cannot practise skills in her restricted home life, she has developed motor delay. This mother needs psychological support and help from social services. The child may require temporary fostering if no other family member can support the mother.

## A boy who is not walking

A family comes to the general paediatric clinic because their 24-month-old son is still not walking. He initially crawled and now bottom-shuffles.

## Differential diagnosis

The move from crawling to bottom-shuffling is unusual and should be considered a form of developmental regression.

The differential diagnosis includes:

- rickets
- hypothyroidism
- muscular dystrophy
- neurometabolic conditions
- neurocutaneous conditions
- myasthenia gravis

## Further information

The boy is not dysmorphic. He scribbles with a colouring pencil and turns pages two at a time. He says two-word sentences. He has very bulky calf muscles and cannot get up from a sitting position. When lifted up, however he can stand steadily and cruise around the furniture. He has an exaggerated lumbar lordosis. His legs are not bowed.

## Conclusion

This child has Duchenne's muscular dystrophy. Blood tests reveal a creatine kinase level of 8000 U/L, and the diagnosis is confirmed on genetic screening.

## A girl with speech delay

A family is referred to the paediatric clinic by the GP. The parents are concerned because their daughter is 30 months old and not saying any words.

## Differential diagnosis

The main causes of speech delay are:

- bilingual household
- neglect
- deafness (congenital and acquired)
- cerebral palsy
- autism spectrum disorder (page 270)
- cleft palate
- bulbar palsy

## Further information

The girl is the first child of parents with normal hearing. She was born at 34 weeks' gestation following a spontaneous onset of labour. There were no neonatal concerns, although she received antibiotic prophylaxis (gentamicin and penicillin) for 48 hours after birth. She did not require phototherapy for jaundice.

Her gross and fine motor development have been normal, and she walked at 11 months.

## Developmental assessment

She does not appear dysmorphic. She makes babbling sounds and says 'Dada' and 'Baba'. She runs stably and will kick a ball. She is very interested in people and objects, and watches people intently as they speak. If handed a pencil, she will scribble. If asked to collect a pencil that is hidden under the table she does not do so, and plays on her own instead. When her name is called from behind a screen, she does not turn to look.

## Conclusion

The reason for her speech delay is deafness. This diagnosis is confirmed on formal audiology testing. This could be genetic, or due to congenital cytomegalovirus infection or ototoxicity caused by gentamicin.

# 5.2 Developmental milestones

The acquisition of a key performance skill is referred to as a milestone. Different milestones are reached at different average ages (**Table 5.1**). Furthermore, the magnitude of the normal age range for attaining each milestone varies widely. You should therefore learn which milestones are consistent (i.e. have a narrow age range that applies to every child, e.g. smiling) and which are inconsistent (i.e. have a wide age range or are not achieved by some children, e.g. crawling).

The developmental milestones also have an absolute age limit by which they should be reached; failure to achieve them is a red flag indicating the need for referral to the developmental clinic for assessment (**Table 5.2**). For example, a child will

| Average age | Fine motor and vision | Gross motor | Social skills | Speech and hearing |
|---|---|---|---|---|
| 6 weeks | Fixes and follows, initially through 45° degrees and then 90° (see **Figure 5.1**); closed hands | Head lag on pull to sit; holds head in line on ventral suspension (see **Figure 5.2**) | Smiles at parent's face | Quietens in response to sound |
| 3 months | Fixes and follows through 180°; hands open; beginning to bring hands to midline | No head lag on pull to sit (see **Figure 5.3**); raises head to 90° when prone | Social smiling (realises smiling makes another person smile in response) | Turns head to sound; coos in response |
| 5–6 months | Voluntary grasp of objects; brings objects to mouth; transfers objects from hand to hand | Rolls from front to back; sits with support | Holds bottle when feeding; looks for removed objects (object permanence) | Turns in response to name; babbles |
| 8–10 months | Pokes at objects with finger; progresses from ulnar to pincer grasp | Sits unsupported; starts to crawl; pulls to stand | Waves bye-bye; finger feeds | Babbles using two-syllables; shouts |
| 12 months | Bangs bricks together; throws objects | Cruises between objects; walks | Claps hands; displays stranger awareness | Says 'Mama' and 'Dada'; understands simple sentences |
| 15 months | Uses pincer grip for small objects | Walks stably | Points and pulls, drinks from a cup | Jabbers; repeats words; understands words for some objects |

**Table 5.1** Developmental milestones. *Continues overleaf*

| 18 months | Scribbles; turns two or three pages of a book at a time; builds a tower of two or three cubes | Carries toys while walking; runs unstably | Holds a cup in both hands; feeds self | Points to named body parts and common objects (e.g. 'door'); follows one-step requests |
|---|---|---|---|---|
| 2 years | Turns pages of a book singly; copies a line | Runs stably | Plays alone; eats with a fork and spoon | Says two-word sentences; has a 50-word vocabulary |
| 2.5–3 years | Builds a tower of six to eight cubes; copies a circle; builds a 'bridge' out of three cubes | Climbs stairs one at a time; kicks a ball | Begins toilet training; puts on shoes and underwear | Says three- or four-word sentences; follows two-step requests |
| 3.5–4 years | Builds a tower of nine or 10 cubes; draws a person with arms and legs; copies a square | Pedals a tricycle; jumps well; hops | Eats with a knife and fork; toilets self unassisted | Asks lots of 'why?' questions; counts to 10; uses the past tense |
| 5 years | Copies a triangle; writes own name; does up buttons | Stands on one foot; comes down stairs one at a time | Chooses own friends; role plays | Counts to 20 |

Table 5.1 *Continued*

probably be walking at around 12 months of age, and ought to be walking by 18 months.

The developmental assessment aims to establish whether a child's progress is:

- normal – developmental milestones are achieved within a recognised time frame
- delayed – there is slower than normal acquisition of skills
- regressing – the child is no longer able to perform skills they once could

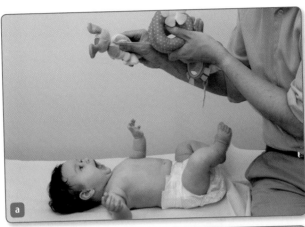

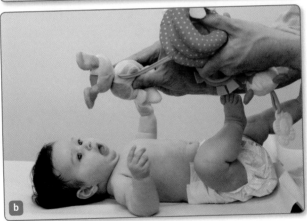

**Figure 5.1** The child is (a) fixing on an object, and (b) following the object through 45°.

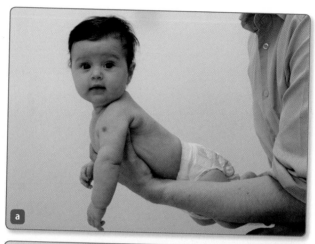

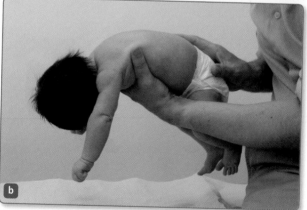

**Figure 5.2** (a) A 3-month-old holds the head in line in ventral suspension, whereas (b) a neonate cannot.

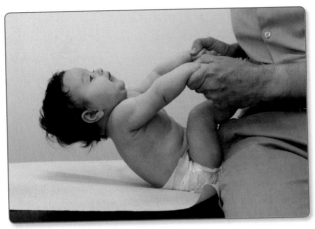

**Figure 5.3** A pull to sitting shows there is no head lag.

| Age | Gross motor | Fine motor | Social | Speech/hearing |
|---|---|---|---|---|
| Any age | Hypotonia, asymmetry of movement | Asymmetry of movement, visual impairment | Unusual eye contact | Hearing loss |
| 5 months | | Not holding object placed in hand | | |
| 6 months | | Not reaching for objects | | |
| 12 months | Not sitting independently | | | |
| 18 months | Not walking | | | No speech. No gestures |
| 2 years | Only walking on tiptoes | Not pointing to share interest | Not pointing to share interest | |
| 2.5 years | Not running | | | |

**Table 5.2** Developmental red flags: urgent investigation is required if present

## 5.3 Common presentations

There are three common presentations to the developmental clinic:

- developmental delay
- developmental regression
- an established diagnosis that requires developmental follow-up

### Delay versus regression

Developmental delay is the slower than expected achievement of new skills. It is either serious or benign and is initially followed up conservatively with monitoring. Developmental regression is the loss of previously acquired skills and should always be taken very seriously. It usually signifies a degenerative progressive pathology that needs prompt investigation.

Causes of delay and regression overlap and include benign, reversible and irreversible causes (**Table 5.3**).

### Benign constitutional delay

As with growth or pubertal delay, some people fall outside the standard deviations of normal development without any

| Category | Example diagnoses |
|---|---|
| Benign constitutional | Familial delay, bottom-shuffling |
| Reversible | Hypothyroidism, nutritional deficiencies (rickets, anaemia), neglect <br> Some visual and auditory problems |
| Progressive | Neurometabolic, neurocutaneous <br> Neglect |
| Global | Global delay, learning difficulties <br> Genetic syndrome <br> Neurometabolic |
| Focal | Dyslexia, dyspraxia |
| Pervasive | Autism spectrum disorder |

**Table 5.3** Causes of developmental delay and regression

underlying pathology. This is usually familial – grandparents are a useful resource in confirming the diagnosis.

*Clinical features*  The child is otherwise well. Delay is usually just in one domain. The most common clinical manifestation is 'bottom-shuffling', in which the child does not crawl and walks late, instead moving around by shuffling in a sitting position. This should be considered a normal variant and only requires reassurance.

## Sensory problems

Without appropriate sensory inputs from vision or hearing, the development of coordinated movement or language skills is extremely difficult.

*Clinical features*  When children with hearing difficulties are not able to pick up visual cues, they will not respond well, or at all, to soft sounds or their name. They often have advanced attentional skills, attempting to lip read. Visual difficulties manifest as a delay in coordinated grasp, poor attention or eye contact, or difficulty in learning colours.

## Hypothyroidism

Thyroxine regulates the basal metabolic rate. Hypothyroidism results in fatigue, poor memory, attentional problems and low appetite. These affect the ability to rehearse and learn skills.

*Clinical features*  A child who develops hypothyroidism becomes less active, feels cold, sleeps a lot and can gain weight despite a poor appetite.

## Rickets

Painful bowing bones, lethargy and even cardiomyopathy can result from vitamin D deficiency. Each limits development in motor and social function, through pain and inability to rehearse skills.

*Clinical features*  Rickets is diagnosed by a low serum vitamin D level. Osteopenia, resulting in bowing of the legs and pain on walking. There may be wrist swelling and a rachitic rosary – bony nodules at the costochondral junctions.

## Neglect or immobility

Without sufficient nutrition or the opportunity to rehearse skills, development can be significantly delayed or even regress. This also applies to children who have had prolonged hospital admissions and cannot develop motor or social skills because of a lack of mobility or stimulation.

*Clinical features*  A neglected child may appear malnourished or unkempt. They may have an abnormal rapport with their parent. If you suspect neglect, always inform a senior colleague.

## Global delay and learning difficulties

These are descriptive diagnoses; they are very common but often unsatisfying for parents. Much developmental delay is idiopathic and the lack of a precise aetiology is distressing. However, even if no precise cause is identified, therapies can be offered and statements of special educational needs written. These help support the child to achieve a higher potential than otherwise possible.

*Clinical features*  'Global delay' describes developmental delay or arrest in two or more domains. 'Learning difficulties' describes idiopathic delay in learning and cognition.

## Genetic conditions and other congenital syndromes

Congenital syndromes are genetic or acquired and can significantly delay development. Common multi-organ-system syndromes are covered in **Chapter 14**.

*Clinical features*  There may be dysmorphia or microcephaly. Abnormalities of the cardiac, gut and renal systems often point to a congenital cause, and hypotonia can be congenital.

## Muscular dystrophy

In muscular dystrophy, dystrophic ('abnormally grown') muscle fibres arise as a result of a genetic abnormality.

*Clinical features*  The patient suffers from chronic progressive weakness of the skeletal muscles. Affected children may walk later than their peers or present with developmental regression. Age of onset varies with subtype. For example, Duchenne's muscular dystrophy presents in early childhood (2–4 years), but Becker muscular dystrophy presents at age 8–12 years.

## Neurometabolic conditions

Metabolic diseases of glycogen storage, mitochondrial function, fats, vitamin metabolism and the urea cycle significantly affect development, but are beyond the scope of this book.

*Clinical features*  A child with a metabolic disease may have a dysmorphia that becomes more obvious with age. They may present with the incidental finding of an enlarged liver or spleen, or with severe hypoglycaemia during periods of metabolic stress, such as viral infections. A basic neurometabolic screen includes serum ammonia, lactate, acyl carnitines and amino acids, with urinary organic acids.

## Neurocutaneous syndromes

Neurocutaneous syndromes present with neurological abnormalities, developmental abnormalities and skin changes. They include neurofibromatosis and tuberous sclerosis (see Chapter 14).

*Clinical features*  Multiple areas of hyper- or hypopigmentation are a clue to neurocutaneous syndromes. Children regress developmentally if they have multiple seizures or become visually impaired.

## Developmental follow-up

Many infants are born with conditions in which development is predicted to be impaired. Such problems include:

- extreme prematurity
- hypoxic–ischaemic encephalopathy (leading to cerebral palsy – see page 155)
- microcephaly
- trisomies (e.g. Down's syndrome – see page 287)
- genetic and other congenital syndromes (see **Chapter 14**)

These children require regular developmental assessment because the associated problems are broad and very variable. Early intervention from appropriate therapists will not cure the underlying condition but will improve both the pace and final outcome of development.

## 5.4 Developmental assessment

Developmental assessment is the skill of mapping a child's progress against that of an average child of a similar age. Age-appropriate development reflects complex neuronal processes of growth, myelination, pruning and migration. As such, the developmental examination should be considered to be a type of neurological assessment (see **Chapter 9**), but one in which the normal tone and coordination of the child varies according to age.

Development is split into four domains (see page 65). 'Learning and cognition' is usually assessed in schools and nurseries. A sequence for examining the other three domains of development is:

- general inspection
- screening questions
- gross motor skills
- fine motor skills
- communication
- social/activities of daily living
- multidisciplinary information
- investigations

The key to assessing development is to allow the child to demonstrate in turn the skills that they can perform within one developmental domain until a skill is reached that cannot be done.

### General inspection

Take time to look at the child at rest. Look particularly for signs of:

- dysmorphia
- pallor
- malnutrition

- neglect
- sensory problems (hearing aids, cochlear implant or spectacles)
- rapport with the parent

## Environment

A 'child friendly environment' (see page 38) is particularly important for the developmental assessment. There should be a large play mat and many toys including:

- large toys
- figures
- plain building blocks
- paper and pens
- books

## Screening

A general screening for developmental concerns and risk factors for developmental delay should use the following script with the parents:

- 'Do you have any concerns about the way your child is behaving, learning or developing?'
- 'Do you have any concerns about the way they move or use their arms or legs?'
- 'Do you have any concerns about how your child talks and understands what you say?'
- 'Does your child enjoy playing with toys?'
- 'Describe what they do while playing.'
- 'Has your child ever stopped doing something they could previously do?'
- 'Does your child get along with others?'
- 'Do you have any concerns about how your child is learning to do things for themself?'

> **Clinical insight**
>
> Parents often have videos of their children performing skills or behaving abnormally, so ask for any videos during screening for developmental delay.

- 'How many languages are spoken at home?'
- 'Is there a history in the family of delayed development?'

Measure the child's height, weight and head circumference.

## Clinical insight

Some children are shy or non-compliant. Continuously ask the parents whether what you are seeing is indicative of their child's abilities. The toddler in front of you who does not want to walk is often able to walk confidently at home.

## Gross motor skills

Run through the gross motor milestones outlined in **Table 5.1**. An older, compliant child can be asked to walk or run, but with younger children you have to be more crafty. Place or hold toys near the child and watch how they reach or approach them.

## Fine motor skills

Select toys of different sizes and see how the child interacts with them. Do they use a one-handed or two-handed approach? Note any hand-preference, which is a 'red flag' for children <3 years old.

Drop a toy and see if the child hunts for it where it has fallen. This is 'object permanence' – an understanding that something which has fallen out of sight has not ceased to exist.

Assess pincer grip by getting the child interested in small objects such as beads or grains of rice.

Make some towers of building block and ask the child to copy you if they can. As a child's fine motor skill improves, the tower of blocks they can build becomes higher. A bridge, although smaller, is a much more complex structure requiring more dexterity and observation than a tower.

Give the child a pen and paper. Draw a line, circle, cross, square and triangle, and ask the child to copy them.

## Communication

- Call the child's name from behind a screen and look at the response.
- Assess eye contact when the child is socially engaged.
- Listen for the use of syllables and words.
- Play naming games with a book or figures – test their knowledge of animals and animal noises.
- Count how many words are in the child's average sentence.

## Social/activities of daily living

You do not have to observe a child to assess this domain. Ask the parents how developed they are in:

- sharing
- stranger awareness
- feeding
- toilet training
- dressing

## Multidisciplinary information

A multidisciplinary approach is by far the best assessment. Look to appropriate therapists for an in-depth assessment of the child's abilities (**Table 5.4**).

### Clinical insight

Children who are brought up in bilingual households are often late developing communication because they are processing two languages at once. To assess their vocabulary, count the same word twice if it is used in both languages. The total number of words the child speaks is often the age-appropriate average.

### Clinical insight

Many activities of daily living require fine motor skills. Be careful not to diagnose global developmental delay in a child for whom an isolated fine motor problem is causing struggles with 'social' skills like dressing or feeding.

| Discipline | Professional |
|---|---|
| Gross motor skills | Physiotherapist |
| Fine motor skills | Occupational therapist<br>Orthoptist/optometrist |
| Feeding | Speech and language therapist<br>Dietitian |
| Speech and language skills | Speech and language therapist<br>Audiologist |
| Social skills | Clinical psychologist |
| Learning and cognition | Educational psychologist, special educational needs co-ordinator at school |

**Table 5.4** The multidisciplinary developmental team

### Investigations

Complete your examination with:

- a cardiac examination (see **Chapter 7**)
- an abdominal examination (see **Chapter 8**)
- a neurological examination (see **Chapter 9**)
- blood tests for nutritional status and genetic syndromes
- a neurometabolic screen (see page 77)

## 5.5 Examination summary

A summary of the developmental examination is given in **Table 5.5**.

| Component | Key findings |
|---|---|
| General inspection | Neglect, dysmorphia, pallor |
| Screening | Developmental concerns, height, weight, head circumference, playing, sharing, family history, languages |
| Gross motor examination | Head movement, sitting, walking, running, climbing |
| Fine motor examination | Grasp, pincer grip, building blocks, drawing |
| Communication examination | Syllables, words, sentences, fluency, languages |
| Social skill examination | Smiling, waving, shyness, feeding, toilet training, independence, pretend |
| Multidisciplinary assessment | See **Table 5.4** |
| Further investigation | Heart sounds, liver size, genetics, nutritional bloods, neurometabolic screen |
| Have you ruled out … ? | Neglect, syndromes, reversible causes |

**Table 5.5** Summary of the developmental examination

## chapter 6

# The respiratory system

The lungs have a limited repertoire of responses to disease: cough, breathlessness and wheeze. Respiratory problems in children often have an infectious cause, and in susceptible children infections can trigger wheezing. Wheezing in other children frequently results from inhalation of a substance, such as pollen or traffic fumes that most people can inhale without problems. A common and serious genetic cause of lung pathology – as well as a shortened lifespan – is cystic fibrosis, most commonly seen in white populations.

The probable diagnoses of respiratory illness depend on the age of the child:

- Babies are likely to have pneumonia or bronchiolitis.
- Toddlers have sometimes inhaled a foreign body.
- Older children are likely to have asthma.

## 6.1 Clinical scenarios

### Poor feeding

A 3-month-old girl is brought in by ambulance from a nearby GP surgery. She has been unwell with a snuffly nose for 2 days, and today she has been able to breastfeed for only 2 minutes at a time because she has been getting out of breath. Her mother thinks that at one point she might have stopped breathing for about 10 seconds.

#### Differential diagnosis

This includes:

- nasal obstruction
- bronchiolitis
- heart failure
- sepsis

#### Further information

On examination, the airway is patent, oxygen saturation is 92% on breathing air, respiration rate is 60 breaths per minute and there are stark chest recessions. Auscultation demonstrates bilateral soft crackles with patchy wheezing. The baby is afebrile. Cardiovascular status is normal. A capillary blood gas shows a pH of 7.35 with a $P\text{CO}_2$ of 5.5 kPa.

## Conclusion

This is the classical presentation of acute bronchiolitis, a viral lower respiratory tract infection that affects babies <1 year of age. Although there is no formal treatment, many babies need admission for supportive care in hospital. The $P\text{CO}_2$ is normal despite significant respiratory distress, so ventilatory support with continuous positive airway pressure (CPAP) is not currently required. The child is admitted for oxygen delivery via a nasal cannula and nasogastric feeding until the respiratory distress subsides.

## Noisy breathing

A 3-year-old boy is rushed into hospital by his parents, who are worried that he has developed very noisy breathing. He seems happy but is making a constant rasping noise when he breathes in. He also has a very loud cough and mild intercostal recession. His mother says that this started with a cold 2 days ago but that he has suddenly deteriorated.

## Differential diagnosis

This child has presented with stridor. The differential diagnosis includes:
- croup
- inhaled foreign body
- laryngomalacia
- epiglottitis
- tonsillitis

## Further information

The boy is playful and happily engaged with a toy, but there is stridor at rest and mild intercostal recession. Oxygen saturations are 95% on breathing air. There is mildly decreased air entry on auscultation and a mild expiratory wheeze. There is no fever, and other observations are normal. The Westley score (see pages 85–86) is 4.

## Conclusion

This boy has mild to moderate croup. Oral dexamethasone should be given and the child observed in the emergency department. If the stridor disappears within 4 hours, the boy can be discharged. If the corticosteroid does not improve the airway obstruction, admission and nebulised adrenaline/epinephrine may be needed to prevent deterioration.

# 6.2 Common presentations

Respiratory illnesses often present in the acute setting as tachypnoea and respiratory distress (see **Table 3.2**), or apnoeas. This is often accompanied by an altered noise of breathing, which many parents describe as a 'wheeze'. The type of noise gives valuable clues to the part of the respiratory tract that is affected. The key presentations in paediatrics are:

- stridor
- wheeze
- cough

## Stridor

Stridor is a gasping or snoring noise made on inspiration that is caused by narrowing of the upper airway. The key differential diagnoses are:

- croup
- inhaled foreign body
- laryngomalacia
- epiglottitis
- tonsillitis

## Croup

Croup (or laryngotracheobronchitis) is caused by a viral infection of the larynx. The swollen airways narrow, so the laminar airflow is disrupted and the airflow becomes turbulent and noisy.

*Clinical features*   There is inspiratory stridor and (as a result of the swollen vocal cords) a harsh 'barking' cough. The Westley score (**Table 6.1**) is used to classify croup.

| Feature | Severity | Score (points) |
|---|---|---|
| Stridor | None | 0 |
| | Only when active/agitated | 1 |
| | At rest | 2 |
| Respiratory distress (e.g. intercostal recession) | None | 0 |
| | Mild | 1 |
| | Moderate | 2 |
| | Severe | 3 |
| Air entry on auscultation | Normal | 0 |
| | Mildly reduced | 1 |
| | Severely reduced | 2 |
| Cyanosis | None | 0 |
| | Only when active/agitated | 4 |
| | At rest | 5 |
| Consciousness | Normal | 0 |
| | Altered | 5 |
| A score of 0–3 is mild, 4–6 moderate, ≥7 severe. | | |

**Table 6.1** The modified Westley scoring system for croup

## Inhaled foreign body
Small children often explore objects with their mouths. Small objects can become lodged in the airway if they are inhaled (aspirated).

*Clinical features* If the aspiration is not witnessed, the clue in the history is a sudden onset of coughing, distress and stridor.

## Laryngomalacia
Laryngomalacia occurs when the cartilaginous walls of the upper airway are not strong enough so collapse inwards on inspiration. This causes turbulent airflow and hence a soft inspiratory stridor.

*Clinical features*  The soft inspiratory stridor may be constant or intermittent. The noise may be louder if the child cries as they take bigger breaths. When the child is asleep, muscle tone in the airway decreases and therefore the stridor is also louder.

## Clinical insight

Do not examine a child with epiglottitis: there is a risk of causing airway obstruction if the child is not kept calm. The child needs urgent intubation by an anaesthetist. Examination, blood tests and antibiotic administration can be done after stabilisation on a ventilator.

### Epiglottitis

Epiglottitis is a bacterial infection of the epiglottis, caused by *Haemophilus influenzae*. It is now rare owing to vaccination.

*Clinical features*  The child with epiglottitis looks very unwell, is flushed, drools and sits with their head forwards to maintain airway patency.

### Wheeze

Wheeze is described as a 'musical' sound that emanates from the chest on expiration. It is sometimes heard at the bedside. Wheeze is caused when airway narrowing disrupts airflow in the lungs.

Not everything that wheezes is asthma. For example, an inhaled foreign body narrows the airways, as does inhalation of a noxious substance, as in glue-sniffing. The more common differential diagnoses are age-dependent:

- bronchiolitis, in infants up to 1 year of age
- virus-induced wheeze, in children aged between 1 and 4 years
- asthma, in older children

### Bronchiolitis

Bronchiolitis is a viral lower respiratory tract infection that occurs in babies and children up to 1 year of age. All respiratory viruses cause it, the most common being respiratory syncytial virus. The symptoms begin with coryza (a runny nose) and low-grade fever. The infection spreads to the bronchioles, which become oedematous and filled with mucus, causing respiratory distress and a wet cough.

*Clinical features* There is visible respiratory distress, with periods of apnoea in more severe cases. Babies struggle with feeding and may vomit from protracted coughing. Auscultation reveals widespread variable crackles and wheezing. The illness is usually worst between day 3 and day 5. It lasts for about 10 days, although the cough may persist for weeks afterwards.

> **Clinical insight**
>
> Croup is caused by a virus, so it is possible to have croup and virus-induced wheeze at the same time.

### Virus-induced wheeze

Virus-induced wheeze is a viral lower respiratory tract infection that occurs in infants between the ages of 1 and 4 years. It presents with an asthma-like response to coughs and colds, but the underlying pathology is different.

*Clinical features* There is cough and coryza, but the main features are wheezing and respiratory distress.

### Asthma

The airway in asthma is hyperreactive to antigens that are normally innocuous (e.g. pollen or animal fur). Inflammation of the small airways causes turbulent airflow, which is heard as wheeze. It also triggers coughing, particularly at night, as dust settles and serum cortisol levels drop.

Asthma may be diagnosed as early as 3 or 4 years of age, if there is a clear trigger. The first sign of asthma may be nocturnal coughing or wheeze exacerbations. Some asthma is exercise induced.

*Clinical features* Unlike bronchiolitis, the wheeze and respiratory distress of asthma (and viral wheeze) is characterised by reversibility with beta-2 agonist inhalers, like salbutamol. These are administered to children via spacer devices (**Figure 6.1**).

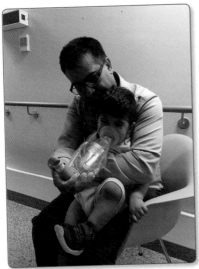

**Figure 6.1** A child using a spacer device. The child's age determines which face mask or mouthpiece is selected.

## Cough

Cough is a very non-specific symptom and results from any pathology at any site in the respiratory tract. Key features of a cough are listed in **Table 6.2**.

### Pneumonia

Pneumonia is an infection of the lung parenchyma and alveolar spaces. The cause is usually viral but sometimes bacterial. A pleural effusion (fluid in the pleural space between the lung and chest wall) can occur secondary to infection. When this fluid is pus, the effusion is termed an empyema.

*Clinical features*  Pneumonia causes fever and tachypnoea, and there may be dyspnoea. There may also be associated systemic symptoms of infection, such as vomiting and tachycardia. Many younger children present complaining of abdominal pain. Pain on inspiration is a classic sign of pleural inflammation, and

| Type | Underlying problem | Differential diagnosis |
|------|--------------------|-----------------------|
| Dry cough | Upper airway infection | Viral upper respiratory tract infection, croup, pertussis, tonsillitis |
| Wet cough | Oedematous lungs | Heart failure, bronchiolitis |
| Productive/fruity cough | Lower airway infection | Pneumonia (viral or bacterial) |
| Tussive vomiting | Forceful cough | Pneumonia, pertussis, bronchiolitis, viral wheeze |
| Barking cough | Upper airway swelling | Croup, tonsillitis |
| Paroxysmal cough | Whooping cough | Pertussis |
| Nocturnal cough | Dust or pollen allergy | Asthma, gastro-oesophageal reflux |
| Haemoptysis | Forceful cough, bleeding at infection site | Tuberculosis, tonsillitis, pneumonia, pertussis |

**Table 6.2** Types of cough and differential diagnosis

children with an effusion or an empyema often sit with the spine curved towards the side of the effusion.

Auscultation may reveal crackles (crepitations) in the affected area; these are caused by air bubbling through fluid or pus within the lung. A 'stony dull' percussion note with quiet air entry suggests pleural effusion.

### Gastro-oesophageal reflux

Children have a short oesophagus and a weak gastro-oesophageal sphincter. They often lie flat after a large liquid feed, and the stomach contents easily reflux back into the oesophagus and the mouth. This irritates the larynx and causes coughing.

*Clinical features*  A child with gastro-oesophageal reflux has a persistent cough that usually occurs after feeds. There may also be a history of vomiting. Diagnosis is often clinical but is confirmed by a pH study.

## Whooping cough

*Bordetella pertussis* and *Bordetella parapertussis* cause a highly contagious bacterial infection of the respiratory tract that produces a loud paroxysmal and persistent 'whooping' cough. This is also known as the 'hundred day cough' because it can last for >3 months. Treatment with macrolide antibiotics affects personal infectivity, but does not necessarily ameliorate symptoms. Vaccination is offered to young children (page 8) and pregnant women.

*Clinical features*    The initial symptoms are those of a coryzal illness, but this is followed by a strong paroxysmal cough. The cough is unsuppressable and strong enough to cause tussive vomiting, subconjunctival haemorrhages and even rib fractures. Smaller babies may present with apnoeas. There is a significant lymphocytosis.

## Tuberculosis

Tuberculosis (TB) is a granulomatous inflammatory infection caused by *Mycobacterium tuberculosis*. Although TB is commonly thought of as a pulmonary infection, it disseminates (miliary TB): the bacterium causes abdominal infections, meningitis, osteomyelitis (Pott's disease) and necrotising lymphadenitis (scrofula). Its slow reproductive cycle makes it a challenge to culture. However, it is diagnosable by a skin reaction to tuberculin (Mantoux test) and interferon-$\gamma$ release assays.

*Clinical features*    TB presents with a vast array of symptoms that are easily confused with other conditions. Respiratory symptoms suggestive of TB include:

- prolonged cough
- haemoptysis
- night sweats
- lymphadenopathy
- fatigue
- weight loss (TB was known as 'consumption' for this reason)
- clubbing

### Clinical insight

TB infection is much more common in patients who are HIV positive. HIV status must therefore be checked in all children with TB.

Unlike other pneumonias, TB has a preference for consolidating the right upper lobe.

## Habitual cough

A cough that arises out of habit may have its origins in a preceding upper respiratory tract infection. There is no associated airway pathology.

*Clinical features*  A habitual cough is more common in older children and younger adolescents than in young children. It is a dry, non-productive cough and is not associated with objective clinical signs such as wheeze or tachypnoea. It may be very persistent and attract a lot of concern from parents.

# 6.3 Examination of the respiratory system

The paediatric respiratory examination follows the same basic format as in adults. However, if a child is not compliant, you will have to reorder the elements and use any windows of opportunity for auscultation.

A sequence for examining the respiratory system is:

- general inspection
- hands
- head and neck
- chest
- investigations

## General inspection

With children, the examination starts during the history. Most of the respiratory assessment can be done from a distance, while the infant or child is sitting with the parent.

## Exposure

A baby is best examined with them lying supine on an open nappy. Toddlers should sit on a parent's lap for comfort. Ask the parents to remove the child's clothing so you can see signs of respiratory distress.

An older child or adolescent is examined as an adult would be: sitting up on a couch at an angle of 45–60° and undressed to the waist.

## General assessment

Inspect for:
- respiratory distress (see **Table 3.2**)
- respiratory rate (count the number of breaths in 30 seconds and double it)
- demeanour
- height and weight
- colour

> **Clinical insight**
>
> An impaired level of consciousness, which may imply hypoxia, does not always take the form of lethargy: hypoxic or hypercapnic children may be combative or irritable.

## The hands

Look at the hands for the following signs:
- clubbing
- cyanosis
- pulse
- asterixis

### Clubbing

**Appearance**  Clubbing is a swelling at the base of the nail bed. The angle formed by the junction of the nail bed with the skin, which is usually concave, becomes convex (**Figure 6.2**).

**Associated conditions**  Clubbing is associated with chronic hypoxia, usually caused by:
- chronic suppurative lung diseases (e.g. cystic fibrosis)
- chronic lung disease of prematurity

### Cyanosis

Cyanosis is a blue discoloration of the skin caused by increased amounts of deoxygenated blood in the capillaries.

**Appearance**  The fingernails may appear blue or grey. Compare the colour to your own to recognise subtle peripheral cyanosis.

**Associated conditions**  Cyanosis results from any cause of acute or chronic hypoxia, for example:
- severe acute asthma
- pulmonary hypertension
- cystic fibrosis
- complex congenital heart disease

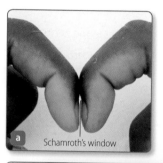

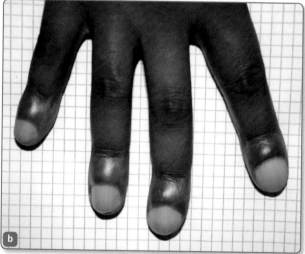

**Figure 6.2** Clubbing of the nails with peripheral cyanosis.

## Pulse

A peripheral assessment of the heart rate and stroke volume should be made.

**Approach** In a baby, feel for the pulse at the brachial artery (medially in the antecubital fossa). In an older child, take the radial pulse. Feel for 30 seconds and double the rate to reach a value for beats per minute.

## Asterixis

Asterixis is a rhythmic flapping movement at the wrists.

**Approach**  Ask the child to hold the arms out straight in front and tip the hands backwards so the palms are facing towards you. If asterixis is present, the hands will 'beat' forwards.

**Associated conditions**  Asterixis is associated with respiratory acidosis (carbon dioxide retention).

## The head and neck

The face and neck can give valuable clues during the respiratory examination. Look at:

- the eyes
- the mouth and tongue
- the lymph nodes

**Approach**  Gently look inside the lower eyelids to assess the colour: they are pale in anaemia. Ask the child to stick out the tongue, and check for cyanosis.

Palpate for lymph nodes in the neck, above the clavicles and in the axillae. Some of these may be raised in TB or viral infections, particularly with Epstein–Barr virus. Nodes may be:

- tender or painless
- fixed or mobile
- limited to one site or distributed in multiple areas

## The chest

Chest examination follows the sequence:

- inspection
- palpation
- percussion
- auscultation

Ensure that you use all four techniques on both the front and back of the chest. The lungs are longer posteriorly than anteriorly, so listening over the back often provides more clues to subtle pathology.

## Inspection

Look for abnormalities of the chest:

- pectus excavatum (sunken sternum)
- pectus carinatum (pigeon/barrel chest)
- scars suggestive of previous surgery (**Figure 6.3**)
- Harrison's sulcus – a subcostal area of indrawn skin with flaring of the ribs at the costal margin; this is the result of chronic increased work of breathing, and is a sign of poorly managed asthma
- a portacath access site under the skin in children who need regular blood tests or intravenous medication (**Figure 6.4**)

## Palpation

**Chest expansion**  Assess chest expansion if hyperexpansion is suspected; this requires a co-operative patient:

> ### Clinical insight
>
> It is difficult to describe in writing the sounds heard in the chest, and it is difficult for a reader to translate even the best-written descriptions into recognisable sounds. Research different chest sounds on the internet: many websites contain useful audio files.

- The examiner places their hands on the front of the child's chest with the fingers pointing upwards (**Figure 6.5**).
- The child is asked to inhale fully and then to exhale; a full expiration should be encouraged.

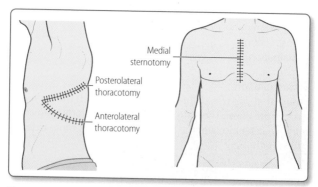

Medial sternotomy

Posterolateral thoracotomy

Anterolateral thoracotomy

**Figure 6.3**  Common sites of scars on chest inspection.

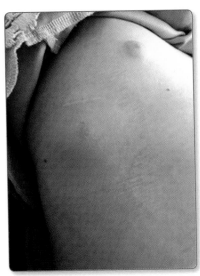

**Figure 6.4** A portacath site. Note the scar and the palpable button under the skin.

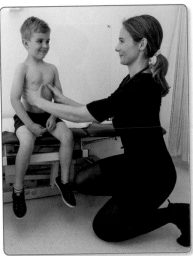

**Figure 6.5** Assessing chest expansion. Note the position of the examiner's thumbs.

- The examiner brings the thumbs together and asks the child to take a full inspiration again; the thumbs should move apart.

### Clinical insight

It is rare to hear sounds of a single pathology. A patient might be coryzal, wheezing and short of breath at the same time. Listen to as many children with simple colds as you can. The bubbling of a snotty nose and rasping of tonsillitis transmit into the chest when you are auscultating.

Unlike in adults, there is not a 'one-size-fits-all' rule for how far apart the thumbs should be by the end of the test. However, it is abnormal if they have barely moved.

### Percussion

Place the middle finger of your non-dominant hand firmly on the child's chest. Then strike the dorsum of that finger with the middle finger of your dominant hand.

Start by percussing the clavicles for a 'reference note'. Then move around the chest, percussing each lung lobe, and comparing (**Figure 6.6**) for:

- areas of dullness (indicating fluid or solid lung – consolidation)

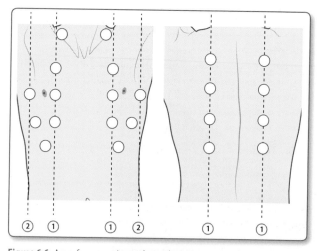

**Figure 6.6** Areas for percussion and auscultation areas over the torso. Dashed lines: ① midclavicular lines; ② midaxillary lines.

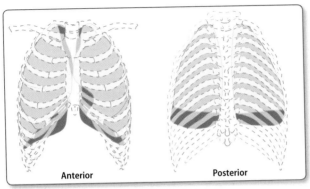

**Figure 6.7** Hyperexpansion. The normal lung borders (blue) are the 6th rib at the front, 8th rib at the side and 10th rib at the back. A lung that has been hyperexpanded by air trapping will have much lower borders (dark pink areas).

- hyperresonance (indicating air in the pleural space)
- hyperexpansion (**Figure 6.7**) – e.g. lung should not be found where you expect a liver

Assess mid-zone pathology by percussing in the axillae.

## Auscultation

Listen to the same areas of the chest (**Figure 6.6**). Compare the two sides  over the front and back, in the axillae (for mid-zone pathology) and in the supraclavicular space (for apical pathology). Note how low down you hear breath sounds to assess whether the chest is hyperexpanded.

**Crackles**   These are caused by air bubbling through fluid – either pus (in infection) or water (in oedema).

**Wheeze**   This is caused by turbulent airflow in the small airways.

**Bronchial breathing**   The whooshing sound of air rushing in and out of the airway is heard, but not the gentler (although louder) noise of the alveoli expanding. Bronchial breathing is heard when the alveoli are not filling with air, because they are collapsed or filled with pus.

**Lack of air entry** This occurs in the following situations:
- collapsed lung
- fluid between the lung and the stethoscope (i.e. an effusion)
- consolidation (i.e. airways full of pus, so that no air can move)
- pneumothorax

These four sounds may be differentiated using percussion and tactile and vocal fremitus. If the lung is consolidated, vocal resonance is increased; if there is a pleural effusion, it is decreased.

## Finishing the examination

Palpate the abdomen: the liver may be displaced downwards by hyperexpanded lungs. It is usual to feel a 1 cm liver edge in babies and infants.

| Component | Key findings |
|---|---|
| General inspection | Weight, height, demeanour<br>colour, respiratory rate and effort, cough and huff |
| Hands | Fingernails (clubbing), asterixis |
| Head and neck | Anaemia, central cyanosis, lymphadenopathy |
| Chest inspection | Deformities, scars |
| Chest palpation | Expansion |
| Chest percussion | Hyperexpansion, dullness (fluid), hyperresonance (pneumothorax) |
| Chest auscultation | Crackles, wheeze, stridor, bronchial breathing, transmitted upper airway noises |
| Abdomen | Hepatomegaly |
| Investigations | Oxygen saturation<br>Peak flow |
| Have you ruled out … ? | Heart failure, airway obstruction, sepsis, tuberculosis |

**Table 6.3** Summary of the paediatric respiratory examination

### Relevant investigations

Simple bedside tests carried out as part of a respiratory examination are:

- saturation monitoring
- peak flow monitoring

Learn how to show a child how to use a peak flow meter by observing their use in clinic or on the wards. Compare the results with the charts showing a 'best predicted value for height'.

## 6.4 Examination summary

A summary of the respiratory examination is given in **Table 6.3**.

# The cardiovascular system

Approximately 8 per 1000 liveborn babies have a congenital cardiac disease. Antenatal fetal scanning detects a significant number of these anomalies, so although they are relatively common, they rarely present unsuspected after delivery.

In utero, blood is oxygenated in the placenta, so there is significantly reduced fetal pulmonary circulation; the lungs are collapsed. Blood travels from the right to the left side of the fetal heart via the ductus arteriosus and foramen ovale (**Figure 7.1a**), and not the lungs. During a baby's first breath, the lungs expand and the pulmonary circulation opens (**Figure 7.1b**) and normal cardiopulmonary physiology takes over. The ductus arteriosus closes over the first week of life.

Cardiac disease presents in a variety of ways, depending on the child's age. Cyanosis and acute deterioration are examples. In addition, seemingly healthy newborns frequently present with heart murmurs which need to be investigated in case they are indicative of congenital cardiac disease.

Older children are less likely to present with structural defects. However, some develop electrophysiological, muscular or infective disorders that affect cardiac output.

## 7.1 Clinical scenarios

### Murmur

A 5-year-old girl attends the emergency department with an allergic reaction to strawberries. There is a widespread urticarial rash and mild tachycardia. Although she is crying and clearly very itchy, she is otherwise well. There is no lip swelling and her blood pressure is at the upper limit of normal. On auscultation, there is a soft systolic murmur.

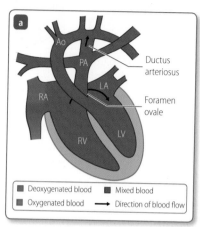

**Figure 7.1** (a) The right-to-left shunt through the fetal ductus arteriosus. (b) The left-to-right shunt through the patent ductus arteriosus of a newborn; this usually closes within a week of birth. Ao, aorta; LA, left atrium; LV, left ventricle; PA, pulmonary artery; RA, right atrium; RV, right ventricle.

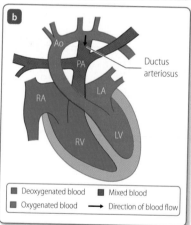

### Differential diagnosis

This includes:

- a pathological murmur, caused, e.g. by a coarctation, ventricular septal defect (VSD) or pulmonary stenosis
- an innocent 'flow murmur' relating to the tachycardia

## Further information

The murmur is soft, located at the left sternal edge and does not radiate. It changes with respiration and posture. Both heart sounds are normal, with intermittent splitting of the second heart sound. Oxygen saturation in the right arm and right leg is 99% on breathing air. There are no features of Turner's syndrome (see page 288).

## Conclusion

The girl probably has an innocent murmur, more pronounced because of the tachycardia. The mother can be reassured, and the allergic reaction treated with chlorpheniramine. The GP should be asked to follow the child up in 2 weeks to ensure that the murmur has disappeared. If it persists, referral to a paediatric cardiology clinic is recommended for possible echocardiography.

## A boy who collapsed playing football

A 9-year-old boy is brought to the emergency department by ambulance after collapsing during a football match. His games teacher performed cardiopulmonary resuscitation and the boy recovered very quickly. He is now tired but says that he 'feels fine'.

## Differential diagnosis

This includes:

- syncope ('fainting')
- arrhythmia
- ventricular outflow tract obstruction (e.g. aortic stenosis)
- cardiomyopathy
- pericarditis
- neurological causes, e.g. seizures (see **Chapter 9**)

## Further information

No seizure was witnessed. The boy has not been feeling unwell and he had no presyncopal symptoms such as dizziness, faintness, nausea or visual disturbance.

Examination shows nothing abnormal. There are no murmurs, which makes a congenital anatomical defect unlikely.

There is no pericardial rub, which makes pericarditis less likely. An ECG shows a corrected QT interval of 490 ms.

### Conclusion

The boy has long QT syndrome, which makes him susceptible to arrhythmias, especially when the heart is stressed. Other family members should be screened with an ECG, and the boy should be referred to a paediatric cardiologist.

## A breathless baby

A 5-day-old baby is brought to the resuscitation area of the emergency department with tachypnoea, tachycardia, cyanosis and marked respiratory distress. Oxygen saturation in the right arm is 79% on breathing air and does not improve with oxygen.

### Differential diagnosis

This includes:

- sepsis
- bronchiolitis (see page 87)
- pneumonia (see page 89)
- heart failure
- congenital heart disease

### Further information

The chest is clear. There is a systolic heart murmur and saturation in the left arm is 88% in 15 L/min oxygen.

### Conclusion

The significant findings are low oxygen saturation in the right arm that do not respond to inhaled oxygen, and higher oxygen saturation in the left arm. These suggest that oxygenated blood is flowing from the pulmonary artery into the aorta via the ductus arteriosus. This is characteristic of duct-dependent cyanotic heart disease. A continuous infusion of prostaglandin E should be started immediately to prevent the duct closing before urgent cardiac surgery can be organised.

## 7.2 Common presentations

Common cardiovascular presentations include:

- heart murmur
- cyanotic baby
- heart failure
- palpitations
- collapse

### Clinical insight

Chest pain is a rare presentation of cardiac disease in children. It may be a presenting symptom of pericarditis, but is more likely to be acid reflux or musculoskeletal pain.

### Heart murmurs

Heart murmurs (**Table 7.1**) are caused by turbulent blood flow:

- through a normal anatomy under mild stress (innocent murmur)
- through a normal anatomy at high volumes [e.g. atrial septal defect (ASD)]
- through a narrowed passage (e.g. pulmonary stenosis or coarctation)
- through an abnormal aperture (e.g. VSD)

| Site of loudest volume | Timing | Radiation | Causes |
|---|---|---|---|
| Apex | Pansystolic | To the axilla | VSD, mitral prolapse |
| Lower left sternal edge | Early systolic | Does not radiate | Innocent murmur |
| Pulmonary area | Pansystolic Ejection systolic | To the back | PDA, AVSD, pulmonary stenosis |
| Pulmonary area | Systolic with split second sound | To the back | ASD |
| Aortic area | Ejection systolic | To the carotid arteries, to the back | Coarctation of the aorta, aortic stenosis |

ASD, atrial septal defect; AVSD, atrioventricular septal defect; PDA, patent ductus arteriosus; VSD, ventricular septal defect.

**Table 7.1** Heart murmurs by location

- in the wrong direction through an incompetent valve (e.g. mitral valve prolapse)
- through a patent ductus arteriosus (PDA)

### Atrial septal defect

In atrial septal defect (ASD) there is a defect between the atria that allows blood to cross from the high-pressure (left) side to the low-pressure (right) side, overfilling the right atrium.

*Clinical features*  The murmur is usually a pulmonary flow murmur caused by the increased volume of blood in the right side of the heart. This increased volume takes longer to expel, so the pulmonary valve closes late; this results in a fixed splitting of the second heart sound (S2).

### Ventricular septal defect

VSD is the most common congenital cardiac defect (30%). Between the ventricles there is a defect that allows blood to cross from the high-pressure (left) side to the low-pressure (right) side (**Figure 7.2**). If the defect is large enough, this shunting of blood overflows the pulmonary circulation.

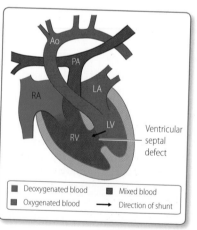

**Figure 7.2** Ventricular septal defect. Ao, aorta; LA, left atrium; LV, left ventricle; PA, pulmonary artery; RA, right atrium; RV, right ventricle.

*Clinical features*  Small VSDs may be asymptomatic and only picked up as a murmur. Larger VSDs sometimes present with heart failure at around 6 weeks of age. The pressure in the right ventricle drops over the

> ## Clinical insight
>
> As the diameter of a tube narrows, the turbulence of the fluid flowing through it increases (think of putting a finger over a tap). Heart murmurs are often softer in large VSDs and become louder as they begin to close.

first 6 weeks of life as the pulmonary vasculature relaxes. This gradually increases the magnitude of the left-to-right shunt, and therefore the volume of the heart murmur. Babies therefore require a second neonatal check at 6 weeks of age (see **Chapter 2**).

Smaller VSDs can be left to close on their own but larger ones require surgical intervention.

## Patent ductus arteriosus

If the ductus arteriosus (see **Figure 7.1b**) remains open past the first few days of life, blood can flow from the high-pressure aorta into the low-pressure pulmonary circulation. PDA is more common in infants who have been born prematurely.

A continuous 'rumbling thunder' murmur is heard, and there may be periodic oxygen desaturation and apnoea. Medication can be given to close the duct (e.g. ibuprofen). If this does not happen, surgical ligation is required.

## Coarctation of the aorta

Coarctation of the aorta (**Figure 7.3**) is caused by narrowing of the aorta, usually where the ductus arteriosus inserts into it.

*Clinical features*  Coarctation is sometimes diagnosed following an incidental detection of a characteristic ejection systolic murmur (see **Table 7.1**). The narrowed aorta results in reduced perfusion of the lower body compared with the upper body. Therefore the cardinal clinical sign of coarctation is weak femoral pulses, with lower blood pressures in the legs than the arms.

In neonates, coarctation of the aorta may present as heart failure (see page 113). Older children may present with hypertension.

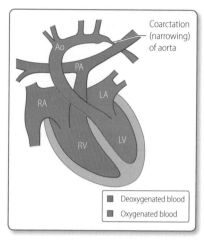

**Figure 7.3** Coarctation of the aorta. Ao, aorta; LA, left atrium; LV, left ventricle; PA, pulmonary artery; RA, right atrium; RV, right ventricle.

| Valve disease | Associated disorders |
|---|---|
| Coarctation | Turner's syndrome |
| Mitral valve prolapse | Marfan's syndrome |
| Mitral stenosis | Rheumatic fever |
| Pulmonary stenosis | Williams' syndrome, Noonan's syndrome |
| Aortic stenosis | Bicuspid aortic valve, rheumatic fever |
| Bacterial colonies | Endocarditis |

**Table 7.2** Types of childhood valve disease

## Clinical insight

If there is suspicion of bacterial endocarditis, test the urine for blood because small deposits of bacteria in the kidneys may cause microscopic haematuria.

### Valve defects

Valve defects are very rare in children. They are either congenital or arise from other pathologies (**Table 7.2**).

### Cyanotic newborn

Oxygen saturation at birth is around 60% but should rise to 95% within the first 10 minutes of life (see **Chapter 2**). In the absence of a respiratory cause for the cyanosis, there is very likely to be a significant congenital cardiac defect. Complex congenital heart diseases are associated with many genetic syndromes (see **Chapter 14**).

## Cyanotic heart disease

Abnormal cardiac anatomy results in mixing of venous and arterial blood.

*Clinical features*  The infant is cyanosed and usually has a murmur. The ductus arteriosus may be the only means of oxygenating blood (as in tetralogy of Fallot) or perfusing the body with oxygenated blood [(as in transposition of the great arteries (TGA)], As the ductus arteriosus closes over the first week, there is worsening:

- hypoxia
- tachycardia
- shock
- lactic acidosis

> ### Clinical insight
>
> Newborn infants who become cyanosed or shocked must be immediately assessed for a duct-dependent cardiac defect. The administration of oxygen to address the hypoxia will accelerate the closure of the duct so prostaglandin E should be started as soon as possible to keep it open.

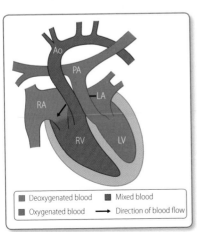

**Figure 7.4** Transposition of the great arteries. In this case, oxygenated blood can only enter the systemic circulation by entering the right side of the heart and mixing with deoxygenated blood via a patent foramen ovale. Ao, aorta; LA, left atrium; LV, left ventricle; PA, pulmonary artery; RA, right atrium; RV, right ventricle.

■ Deoxygenated blood    ■ Mixed blood
■ Oxygenated blood    ⟶ Direction of blood flow

### Transposition of the great arteries

In TGA, the aorta and pulmonary trunk arise from the wrong ventricles (**Figure 7.4**). Unless there is also an ASD or PFO, the only way for oxygenated blood to enter the systemic circulation is via the ductus arteriosus.

### Total anomalous pulmonary venous drainage

The pulmonary veins drain into the vena cava instead of the left atrium. This results in mixed blood entering the right ventricle. As in TGA, the aortic circulation can only be perfused via an ASD or PDA.

### Tetralogy of Fallot

The four features of tetralogy of Fallot are shown in **Figure 7.5**. It is particularly associated with 22q microdeletion syndrome (see page 292) and Down's syndrome (see page 287).

The outflow tract of the right side of the heart is partially obstructed, owing to the pulmonary stenosis. Some blood, unable to get through the pulmonary valve, will flow from the right ventricle across the VSD or out into the overriding

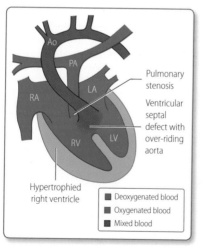

**Figure 7.5** Tetralogy of Fallot. Ao, aorta; LA, left atrium; LV, left ventricle; PA, pulmonary artery; RA, right atrium; RV, right ventricle.

Pulmonary stenosis

Ventricular septal defect with over-riding aorta

Hypertrophied right ventricle

■ Deoxygenated blood
■ Oxygenated blood
■ Mixed blood

aorta. This may only happen sporadically, resulting in intermittent cyanotic spells. In severe stenosis, the only route for blood to flow into the pulmonary circulation is via the ductus arteriosus.

## Atrioventricular septal defect

There is an abnormality in both the atrial and the ventricular septum. Oxygenated and deoxygenated blood mix in the atria and again in the ventricles. Atrioventricular septal defects are associated with Down's syndrome (see page 287).

## Heart failure

Heart failure describes the symptoms and signs that occur when the pumping action of the heart is not capable of expelling the required ventricular output. Fluid 'backs up' in the lungs (left ventricular failure) or the liver and peripheral tissue (right ventricular failure).

In most adult cardiology patients, the heart has two completely separate sides, so a single pathology causes either left- or right-type heart failure. However, most paediatric cardiology patients have defects that interrupt this left/right system. In the presence of a septal defect, for example, blood will shunt from the left side of the heart to the right, overloading the right ventricle, and underperfusing the aorta. This results in a mixed picture of left and right failure.

**Table 7.3** lists the key signs of heart failure in a baby.

| Early | Late |
|---|---|
| Poor feeding | Failure to thrive |
| Poor weight gain | Generalised oedema |
| Tachypnoea, especially during feeds | Ascites |
| Sweating during feeds | |
| Murmur | |
| Fine crackles on auscultation of the chest | |
| Hepatomegaly | |

**Table 7.3** Symptoms and signs of heart failure

## Palpitations and collapse

'Palpitations' are periods of increased awareness of one's own heartbeat. This is usually a benign condition: everyone has this feeling after exercise or when anxious. If, however, these episodes occur with an abnormal heart rhythm (arrhythmia) or episodes of collapse, they require urgent investigation.

## Collapse
### Syncope

Syncope, or 'fainting', occurs when there is a sudden fall in cerebral perfusion pressure or oxygenation. There are many causes:

- dehydration
- hypoglycaemia
- orthostatic hypotension (a drop in blood pressure on standing, seen in Addison's disease)
- panic attack
- medications (e.g. beta blockers)
- drugs and alcohol
- reflex anoxic seizures (breath-holding episodes following a minor injury in toddlers)
- arrhythmias
- left ventricular outflow tract obstruction (e.g. aortic stenosis or coarctation)

*Clinical features*  The classic history is of a presyncopal prodrome of lightheadedness, visual disturbance and pallor. A collapse with loss of consciousness resolves in seconds. During a faint, the patient often has enough presence of mind to collapse in a way that will not hurt them. When consciousness is regained, the patient often feels normal within a few minutes.

### Supraventricular tachycardia

This is caused by an abnormal electrical rhythm in the atria. The atria beat rapidly and, if this rapid impulse is electrically transmitted to the ventricles, the heart will beat at >180 beats per minute. Cardiac output may be decreased because the heart does not have time to refill between beats.

Aberrant electrical pathways in the heart may cause or exacerbate supraventricular tachycardia, as in Wolff–Parkinson–White syndrome.

*Clinical features* There may be palpitations. The prodrome to a collapse includes nausea, changing vision or hearing loss. ECG shows a narrow complex tachycardia, with delta (or 'J') waves in Wolff–Parkinson–White syndrome.

## Long QT syndrome

Long QT syndrome comprises a group of genetic disorders that affect surface membrane ion channels on the cardiac muscle. Children and adults with long QT syndrome can have arrhythmias or cardiac arrests.

*Clinical features* There may be a personal history of fainting and a family history of sudden unexplained death in young people, especially during exertion. The ECG shows a prolonged corrected QT interval of >0.44 s.

## Cardiomyopathy

In cardiomyopathy, the cardiac muscle is weakened, leading to a decrease in the amount of blood that the heart is able to pump. This may cause heart failure.

Common causes include:

- hypertrophic obstructive cardiomyopathy, in which bulky myocardium obstructs the outflow
- viral myocarditis (especially Coxsackie A), which inflames the muscle and decreases its power of contraction
- rheumatic fever (occurring after streptococcal inflammation of the myocardium and valves; see page 192)
- vitamin D deficiency, which results in depletion of myocardial calcium

*Clinical features* Cardiomyopathy usually presents with heart failure (**Table 7.3**) and an enlarged heart on radiography. Myocarditis increases the risk of arrhythmias.

## 7.3 Examination of the cardiovascular system

The paediatric cardiac examination follows the same overall format as that in adults. However, because a child may not be compliant, you may have to restructure the order and use any windows of opportunity for auscultation.

A sequence for examination is:
· general inspection
· hands
· pulses and blood pressure
· head and neck
· heart
· investigations

### General inspection
#### Exposure

Babies should have clothes removed down to the nappy and be examined supine. Most children can be positioned as for adult, lying on a bed at 45° and with clothes removed fully to the waist. Always prioritise the patient's comfort – young children will be much more compliant in their parent's lap (see **Chapter 3**). Adolescent girls should keep their bra on.

#### General assessment
Inspect for:
· dysmorphia
· weight
· head circumference
· colour
· respiratory distress (see page 37)
· scars suggestive of previous surgery (e.g. midline sternotomy from a cardiac reconstruction; left lateral thoracotomy from ligation of a PDA, coarctation repair or Blalock-Taussig shunt; and drain sites)

### Hands
The hands should be examined for:
· clubbing

- splinter haemorrhages
- pulses and blood pressure

## Clubbing

*Appearance*  Clubbing is a swelling at the base of the nail bed (**Figure 7.6**).

*Associated conditions*  The cardiac conditions associated with clubbing are cyanotic congenital heart disease, endocarditis and atrial myxomas.

## Splinter haemorrhages

*Appearance*  These are small linear bleeds underneath the nail.

*Associated conditions*  Splinter haemorrhages are caused by small colonies of bacteria detaching from an infected valve and lodging in the nail bed. They are a sign of endocarditis.

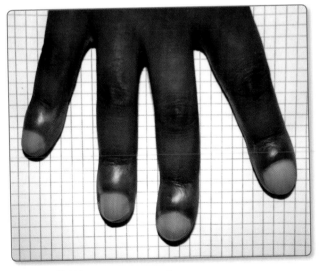

**Figure 7.6** Clubbing.

## Pulses

In a baby or toddler, feel the pulse at the brachial artery. In an older child, check the radial pulse. Examine the pulse for rate, rhythm and volume, and for the brachial–brachial or brachial–femoral delay of coarctation.

## Head and neck

### Eyes

Check the conjunctivae for anaemia (they may be pale), and the sclerae for jaundice. Haemolysis caused by a prosthetic heart valve produces both of these.

### Jugular venous pulse

If the child is able to sit up at 45°, the jugular venous pressure (JVP) should be examined. A raised JVP suggests that right-sided heart pressures are raised.

In a baby, where a short, fat neck makes viewing the JVP impossible, an enlarged liver is the 'examination equivalent' of a raised JVP.

### Mouth and tongue

Look at the underside of the tongue to assess for central cyanosis – a blue discoloration (**Figure 7.7**). Inspect the teeth: poor dentition can be an entry route for bacteria and result in infective endocarditis.

## Precordium

Assess for a visible apex beat.

Palpate for the apex beat. If no apex beat can be felt on the left side, feel on the right side in case there is dextrocardia. Palpate for heaves and thrills; a right ventricular heave will be felt at the left sternal border. Thrills should be palpated for over the corresponding auscultatory valve areas (**Figure 7.8**).

### Clinical insight

An obese child may need to lean forward during auscultation to make the heart sounds audible. This position draws the heart closer to the chest wall and compensates for the muffling effect of subcutaneous fat.

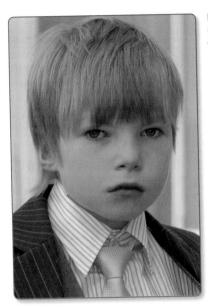

**Figure 7.7** Cyanosis. (note the dusky lips and eyes).

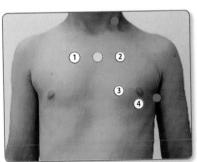

**Figure 7.8** Auscultation areas. Valve areas: ① aortic, ② pulmonary, ③ tricuspid, ④ mitral/apex. Blue spots indicate radiations: axilla, neck, back.

## Auscultation

Auscultation is performed to assess heart sounds and listen for murmurs.

## Heart sounds

Begin by listening at the apex (the 'mitral area') (**Figure 7.8**) to the cycle of heart sounds – 'lub-dub, lub-dub'. The rate is faster than an adult's. As the left main bronchus lies close to the apex, harsh breathing noises interfere with the heart sounds, so do not mistake breath sounds for a heart murmur.

Move systematically through the other three areas (**Figure 7.8)**, listening carefully for abnormal or added sounds. Murmurs should be graded (**Table 7.4**).

***Splitting of the second heart sound*** There are occasionally three, rather than two, heart sounds ('lub-dadub, lub-dub, lub-dadub').

The second heart sound (S2) is made up of the aortic valve closing (the A2 sound) and the pulmonary valve closing (the P2 sound). The timing of the two components varies with breathing. On inspiration, negative intrathoracic pressure draws more blood into the right side of the heart. This increased volume takes longer to cross the pulmonary valve, so the pulmonary valve closes later – P2 occurs after A2. The reverse occurs in expiration.

'Fixed splitting' (where the 'lub-dadub' pattern does not alter with breathing) occurs in an ASD when the right heart is constantly overfilled by flow through the ASD.

Listen in three areas to assess the radiation of murmurs (**Figure 7.8**).

| Grade | Description |
|-------|-------------|
| 1 | Can be heard by an expert in a quiet room |
| 2 | Sounds quiet to a non-expert in a quiet room |
| 3 | Heard easily, but with no added thrill |
| 4 | Heard as loud, with an added thrill |
| 5 | Heard as loud across the entire precordium, with a thrill |
| 6 | Audible without a stethoscope ('heard at the end of the bed') |

**Table 7.4** Grading the intensity of heart murmurs

## Finishing the examination

By the end of the examination, the patient should be leaning forward as you have checked the back for radiating murmurs. Listen to the lung bases for the fine crackles of pulmonary oedema, and press over the sacrum to assess for sacral oedema.

With the patient lying back down, palpate for a liver edge to identify enlargement. The liver may be pulsatile in tricuspid regurgitation as the impulse from the right ventricle is transmitted back through the open tricuspid valve.

Feel the ankles for oedema, and inspect the toenails for clubbing.

## Investigations

Key cardiovascular investigations are:

- oxygen saturation
- blood pressure
- ECG
- Holter monitoring
- echocardiography

> **Clinical insight**
>
> A minimum of 50 g/L of deoxygenated blood needs to be present before cyanosis is clinically recognisable. Therefore a child with anaemia may not appear blue.

### Oxygen saturation

Oxygen saturation should be checked in children who look unwell. In a child with a murmur, oxygen saturation should be recorded in the right arm and at least one other limb to ensure that blood is not flowing through a PDA.

### Blood pressure

Measurement of blood pressure requires a calm child and a correctly sized cuff: the cuff should cover two thirds of the upper arm. Plot the result on a percentile chart to aid interpretation. In children with heart murmurs, check the blood pressure in all four limbs to rule out coarctation of the aorta.

### ECG

The ECG varies throughout childhood. In the first years of life, T wave inversion is normal in leads V1, V2 and V3, but the pattern gradually changes towards an adult pattern as the child ages. Interpretation of paediatric ECGs requires specialist input.

## Holter monitoring

This is 24-hour-long ECG recording using on a monitor worn under the child's clothing. It picks up intermittent arrhythmias and correlates them with the patient's symptoms, such as palpitations or syncopal episodes.

## Echocardiography

This is a dynamic ultrasound test that examines the physical structure of the heart and the velocity of blood flow. It is used to detect anatomical abnormalities, shunts and identify areas of unusual pressure, such as in pulmonary hypertension.

## 7.4 Examination summary

A summary of the cardiovascular examination is given in **Table 7.5**.

| Component | Key findings |
|---|---|
| General inspection | Weight, height, head circumference, colour, respiratory rate and effort |
| Hands | Fingernails (clubbing, splinters), pulses |
| Face | Anaemia, jaundice, central cyanosis |
| Chest inspection | Visible impulses, scars |
| Chest palpation | Apex, heaves, thrills |
| Chest auscultation | Murmur – location, radiation, grade; splitting of heart sounds |
| Back and abdomen | Pulmonary oedema, hepatomegaly, peripheral oedema |
| Investigations | Oxygen saturation, ECG, blood pressure |
| Have you ruled out … ? | Heart failure, complex congenital heart disease |

**Table 7.5** Summary of paediatric cardiovascular examination and associated investigations

# The abdomen

Vomiting, diarrhoea and abdominal pain are among the most common symptoms in children and vary greatly in severity. Each can be a benign result of age or diet, or indicate severe pathology. Distinguishing constipation from Crohn's disease can be more of a challenge in practice than one might think.

Abdominal problems are accompanied by a broad spectrum of parental anxiety, which is not always in proportion to the problem. Patients and parents will have different ideas of what constitutes 'diarrhoea' or 'severe pain'. The key is to listen and understand the family's perspective. Parents who have lived in developing countries are often very worried about vomiting and loose stools because diarrhoea is the biggest killer of children worldwide. It is not reasonable to expect parents familiar with cholera, dysentery or typhoid to be able to distinguish them from enterovirus infection.

Palpation is central to the abdominal examination. Although often nothing abnormal is found, a negative examination does not rule out significant pathology – pay close attention to the history.

## 8.1 Clinical scenarios

### Abdominal pain

A 15-year-old girl comes to the emergency department with her parents. There is a 1-day history of severe abdominal pain, and she has vomited once. There was a loose stool yesterday but the bowels have not been open today. There is pallor and she has a mildly raised heart rate. The girl is unable to sit up on the trolley.

### Differential diagnosis
This includes:
- gastroenteritis
- appendicitis

- ectopic pregnancy
- intestinal obstruction

### Further information

Examination reveals a tender right iliac fossa with guarding, and bowel sounds are absent. The girl's menstrual period has just finished, and she has a regular menstrual cycle. A urinary pregnancy β-human chorionic gonadotropin test is negative. There is no fever, and the vomitus was not bile stained.

### Conclusion

The most likely cause is appendicitis. The specific tenderness in the right iliac fossa is not typical of gastroenteritis, and the recent period and negative urinary β-human chorionic gonado-tropin test make ectopic pregnancy highly unlikely. There is no bile-stained vomitus to suggest a bowel obstruction.

## Chronic diarrhoea

A 3-year-old boy is brought to the GP by his mother. She is concerned because his stools always seem to be loose compared with those of other children. His mother thinks that he has not put on much weight recently.

### Differential diagnosis

The following differential diagnoses should be considered:
- coeliac disease
- cystic fibrosis
- lactose intolerance
- inflammatory bowel disease
- toddler diarrhoea

### Further information

On further questioning, it transpires that the diarrhoea has been present for over a year. The stools are also foul-smelling and difficult to flush away. On examination, the boy is noted to be thin and looks miserable. His records reveal a static weight, and his height velocity is slowing down.

## Conclusion

The clinical features suggest malabsorption as the cause of both the diarrhoea and the failure to gain weight. Toddler diarrhoea does not lead to growth problems, and malabsorption is rare in lactose intolerance. Inflammatory bowel disease is possible but unlikely in this young age group.

Coeliac disease seems to be the most likely cause, but a sweat test is needed to rule out cystic fibrosis.

## 8.2 Common presentations

The key presentations of abdominal conditions include:
- abdominal pain
- vomiting
- diarrhoea
- abdominal mass or distension

### Abdominal pain

Abdominal pain is a very common presentation with a wide differential diagnosis, but this is very quickly pared down using a structured history (**Table 8.1**). The **TENDS** mnemonic (see page 5) is key in establishing a differential diagnosis; the time course of the pain is particularly relevant.

### Constipation

Most constipation results from a combination of dietary factors (e.g. low-fibre diet or inadequate hydration) and psychosocial factors (e.g. a reluctance to defecate in school toilets). A rare cause of constipation is Hirschsprung's disease, in which there is an abnormality in the neuronal development of the intestine.

*Clinical features* There is frequent, intermittent, abdominal pain, decreased frequency of defecation and pellet-like or large-volume stools. If there is severe impaction, liquid stool from above can leak around the blockage; this often stains the underwear and is mistaken for diarrhoea.

Signs on examination may include a mass in the left iliac fossa that can be indented and has the texture of putty.

| Component of history* | Finding | Diagnosis |
|---|---|---|
| Triggers | Dietary | Coeliac disease, lactose intolerance, allergy |
| | Stress | Irritable bowel syndrome, functional pain |
| | Eating | Gastric ulcer, reflux |
| Evolution | With vomiting or diarrhoea | Gastroenteritis, appendicitis, urinary tract infection, obstruction, diabetic ketoacidosis |
| | With bloody diarrhoea | Inflammatory bowel disease, intussusception, cow's milk protein intolerance, Meckel's diverticulum. |
| | With weight loss | Coeliac disease, gastric ulcer, Crohn's disease, diabetes, allergy |
| | Without weight loss | Constipation, functional pain, ulcerative colitis |
| Nature | Colicky | Renal pain, urinary tract infection, gastroenteritis |
| | Dull, central | Constipation, gastroenteritis, diabetes |
| | Upper | Gastritis, ulcer, pneumonia, pancreatitis |
| | Lower | Cystitis, appendicitis, constipation, ulcerative colitis, ectopic pregnancy, torsion of cyst or testis |
| Duration | Acute | Infective causes, intussusception |
| | Chronic (>2 weeks) | Constipation, inflammatory bowel disease, coeliac disease, functional pain |
| Severity | Waking at night | Inflammatory bowel disease |
| | Unable to sit | Peritonism, appendicitis, torsion |
| | Preventing daily activities | Inflammatory bowel disease, abdominal migraine |

*Use the TENDS mnemonic (see page XXX).

**Table 8.1** Common causes of abdominal pain

## Urinary tract infection

The most common cause of urinary tract infections (UTIs) is Gram-negative bacteria, especially *Escherichia coli*. Anatomical abnormalities of the urinary tract predispose to infection,

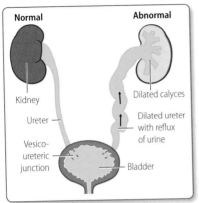

**Figure 8.1** Vesicoureteric reflux.

usually by causing vesicoureteric reflux (**Figure 8.1**).

*Clinical features* Common symptoms of a UTI in children include:
- fever
- a non-specific feeling of being 'unwell'
- nausea and vomiting
- abdominal pain (often suprapubic or loin pain)
- dysuria and urinary frequency
- secondary nocturnal enuresis

Diagnosis is by urine dipstick and culture.

## Clinical insight

Recurrent UTIs can be a sign of anatomical problems. These are visualised using ultrasound, a micturating cystourethrogram or a mercaptoacetyltriglycine (MAG-3) scan. Severe UTIs cause renal damage, which is visualised on a dimercaptosuccinic acid (DMSA) scan. Consult local guidelines to determine which scan is appropriate for your patient, depending on their age.

### Acute appendicitis

Acute appendicitis is the most common surgical cause of an acute abdomen in children.

*Clinical features* The pain classically starts lower down and centrally in the abdomen but then spreads to the right iliac fossa. Children often feel generally unwell with a decreased appetite, nausea and vomiting.

## Intussusception

Intussusception is an uncommon but important cause of acute onset abdominal pain, where part of the bowel telescopes inside itself. This often needs surgical correction.

***Clinical features***  Acute onset severe abdominal pain, which worsens and partially resolves in waves is sometimes accompanied by severe rectal bleeding of 'redcurrant jelly' stools. As symptoms persist, the patient can develop bowel ischaemia, and go into shock. Risk factors include cystic fibrosis, polyps and mesenteric adenitis (inflammation of the abdominal lymph nodes in viral infections).

## Inflammatory bowel disease

Ulcerative colitis and Crohn's disease are inflammatory diseases of the bowel wall with a poorly understood aetiology The diagnosis of inflammatory bowel disease is confirmed by endoscopy and biopsy.

***Clinical features***  Ulcerative colitis is inflammation of the rectum and colon, and therefore presents as chronic abdominal pain and bloody diarrhoea. It is classified using the Paediatric Ulcerative Colitis Activity Index (**Table 8.2**).

Crohn's disease occurs anywhere in the alimentary canal – from mouth to anus – and produces areas of painful ulceration and strictures. Weight loss from malabsorption is common in Crohn's disease (80% of patients), and there are raised inflammatory markers and platelets, and low serum albumin levels.

## Colic

'Colic' is an imprecise term used to describe abdominal discomfort in babies that has no obvious pathological cause. The aetiology is unknown but theories include swallowed air that has not been burped up and instead has passed into the gut, distending it. Colic drops are said to alter the surface tension of the milk to release bubbles more easily, but their effectiveness is not clear and they are only effective alongside good burping techniques.

| Item | Basis for allocating points |
|------|------------------------------|
| Abdominal pain | Whether pain is present and can be ignored or not |
| Rectal bleeding | Frequency and volume |
| Stool consistency | How formed or unformed |
| Stool frequency | Motions per day |
| Nocturnal stools | Do or don't occur |
| Activity | Degree of limitation or restriction |
| Total score: 10–30, mild disease; 35–60, moderate disease; ≥65, severe disease. | |

**Table 8.2** Parameters assessed by the Paediatric Ulcerative Colitis Activity Index. Points are allocated according to a published scale for each item. Disease severity is determined by the total score (e.g. 10–30 is mild and ≥65 is severe disease). Online calculators assist in the appropriate allocation of points in each category.

## Testicular torsion

Torsion occurs when the testis rotates inside the scrotum, occluding the blood supply from the gonadal artery. This causes irreversible necrosis after 6–8 hours; therefore acute testicular pain should be treated as a surgical emergency.

*Clinical features* On examination, the testicle is tender and either sits high or is retracted in the scrotum. A blue discoloration may be visible through the skin. The main differential diagnosis is epididymo-orchitis, which presents in an almost identical way. Blood flow to the testicle is assessed using ultrasound.

## Vomiting

The causes of vomiting can be divided into intracranial, peripheral and gastrointestinal (**Table 8.3**).

Acute vomiting is most commonly caused by a viral infection, such as norovirus. A respiratory infection causing a cough can give rise to post-tussive vomiting.

In young children, a simple fever, and indeed almost any infection of any system, often causes vomiting. Key 'red flags' to look for include:

- persisting vomiting with fever – bacterial meningitis or pyelonephritis

| Causes | Typical associated features |
|---|---|
| **Central causes** | |
| Raised intracranial pressure | Morning headaches |
| Migraine | Aura, flashing lights, headache |
| Brainstem disease | Nystagmus, ataxia |
| **Peripheral causes** | |
| Otitis media | Ear pain, ear discharge |
| Vestibular disease | Dizziness |
| Diabetic ketoacidosis | Raised blood sugar |
| Urinary tract infection | Fever, dysuria |
| Pregnancy | Positive β-human chorionic gonadotropin |
| **Gastrointestinal causes** | |
| Gastroenteritis | Fever, diarrhoea |
| Pyloric stenosis | Presents in a baby, with a palpable mass and projectile vomiting |
| Appendicitis | Right iliac fossa pain |
| Intestinal obstruction | Bile-stained vomitus |

Table 8.3 Causes of vomiting in children and typical associated features

- nocturnal or early morning vomiting (in the absence of cough) – pregnancy or brain tumour
- green vomit – bowel obstruction, e.g. from volvulus

Infants frequently vomit or posset small amounts of milk after feeding, and this is normal.

Two important gastrointestinal causes of vomiting are:
- gastro-oesophageal reflux disease
- pyloric stenosis

## Gastro-oesophageal reflux disease

This is caused by a functionally immature gastro-oesophageal sphincter that allows stomach contents and acid to reflux into the oesophagus. Gastro-oesophageal reflux is a normal phenomenon in babies, whereas gastro-oesophageal reflux 'disease' (where the reflux causes excessive symptoms or demonstrable pathology) should be treated. Most cases are in healthy infants, but infants with a neurological disease such as cerebral palsy can have severe reflux disease. It is less common in older children.

*Clinical features*  The main clinical features that parents describe are:
- posseting and regurgitation
- excessive crying, especially after feeds
- recurrent apnoea
- abnormal neck extension (Sandifer's syndrome)
- distress on being laid flat

## Pyloric stenosis

Pyloric stenosis classically affects boys around the age of 4–8 weeks. It is progressive hypertrophy of the muscle surrounding the pylorus of the stomach, causing gastric outflow obstruction.

*Clinical features*  Infants present with worsening vomiting, eventually vomiting whole feeds every feed. They are hungry babies, with weight loss and signs of dehydration. Blood gas analysis shows a hypokalaemic, hypochloraemic alkalosis.

## Diarrhoea

Diarrhoeal illness is the biggest killer worldwide of children aged <5 years. Patients and parents have widely different ideas of what constitutes diarrhoea, from an increased frequency of normal motions to the passage of persistently liquid stools.

The time course is  essential to diagnosis:
- acute diarrhoea (<2 weeks), commonly resulting from infective gastroenteritis or drugs
- chronic diarrhoea (>2 weeks) (see **Table 8.4**)

The main differential diagnoses of diarrhoea are:
- gastroenteritis
- inflammatory bowel disease (see page 128)

| Type of diarrhoea | Typical features |
|---|---|
| **Malabsorptive diarrhoea** | |
| Coeliac disease | Poor weight gain, lethargy, pallor |
| Cystic fibrosis | Failure to thrive, chest infections |
| Post-gastroenteritis (brush border enzyme deficiency) | Follows acute infection, positive stool reducing substances |
| **Secretory diarrhoea** | |
| Cholera | Occurs in epidemics, profuse watery stools |
| **Inflammatory diarrhoea** | |
| Inflammatory bowel disease (Crohn's disease, ulcerative colitis) | Blood or mucus in stools, abdominal pain |
| Cow's milk protein intolerance | Rashes, atopic family history, blood in stools |

Table 8.4 Causes of chronic diarrhoea in children and typical associated features

- malabsorption
- bloody diarrhoea

### Gastroenteritis

Infectious gastroenteritis is caused by a variety of pathogens. Viruses such as rotavirus are the most common, and bacteria and protozoa less common. Fresh blood in the stool may suggest a bacterial colitis caused by *Escherichia coli*, *Campylobacter* spp. or *Salmonella* spp. Since the introduction of a rotavirus vaccine in 2013, UK hospital admissions for viral gastro-enteritis in the under-1s have fallen by 70%.

### Clinical insight

Percentage dehydration is calculated from the percentage of body weight lost or estimated from the clinical signs. Many parents have a recent weight record for their child. Dehydrated children need their normal fluid maintenance intake plus the percentage dehydration of their body weight in fluid, which may be several litres. Do not simply prescribe 105–110% of normal fluid maintenance, which will be much less than they need. This is a common and dangerous error.

*Clinical features* The main feature is loose stools; this term refers to a liquid consistency of stools or an increased frequency of defecation. Blood in the stools should be noted.

It is vital to assess hydration status. Mild dehydration (<5%) presents with cracked lips, dry skin and a lower than normal urine output.

The clinical features of severe dehydration (>10%) are:
- looking 'unwell'
- decreased energy levels, with lethargy or decreased consciousness
- pale or mottled skin
- cool extremities
- prolonged capillary refill
- absent urine output
- tachycardia
- tachypnoea
- compensated metabolic acidosis
- low blood pressure – a late, very serious sign

## Malabsorption

The common causes of malabsorption are shown in **Table 8.4**.

Treatment of diet-related malabsorption is by temporary withdrawal of dairy products (lactose intolerance is usually transitory) or permanent withdrawal of gluten (coeliac disease is usually lifelong).

### Clinical insight

Raised IgA antibody to tissue transglutaminase (TTG) indicates a diagnosis of coeliac disease. Always check serum immunoglobulins at the same time, because IgA deficiency (low total serum IgA) will produce a falsely reassuring low TTG result. In cases of total IgA deficiency, an intestinal biopsy may be required to confirm the diagnosis by histology.

## Rectal bleeding

Passing small streaks of frank red blood in the stool is common in simple viral gastroenteritis, or in cases of anal fissures and haemorrhoids.

However, passing large volumes of frank red blood is never normal and needs urgent investigation. The differential diagnosis includes:

- bacterial or protozoal infective diarrhoea (page 132)
- ulcerative colitis (page 128)
- Crohn's disease (page 128)
- intussusception (page 128)
- Meckel's diverticulum

## Meckel's diverticulum

Meckel's diverticulum is a common malformation of the intestinal tract found in 2% of the population. It is a vestigial remnant of the omphalomesenteric duct.

*Clinical features*  Meckel's diverticulum is often benign and goes unnoticed through life. However they are prone to bleeding and can cause catastrophic blood loss per rectum when they do. It is diagnosed by technetium-99m scan or laparoscopy and requires surgical removal if bleeding.

## Abdominal masses

Abdominal masses may be normal findings, such as stool or a full bladder, or signify serious disease. A differential diagnosis is shown in **Table 8.5**.

### Inguinal hernia

Infantile inguinal hernias are always indirect and are caused by a patent processus vaginalis, which allows herniation through the deep inguinal ring. The hernia may intermittently contain various abdominal contents, including bowel.

*Clinical features*  Inguinal hernias present with a unilateral or bilateral mass arising from the deep inguinal ring and extending a variable distance, potentially all the way, into the scrotum. If the hernia can be reduced, it often reappears when the child coughs or cries.

Hernias must be differentiated from testicular masses which warrant more urgent investigation. The key difference is that it is possible to get above a testicular mass but not a hernia.

| Abdominal mass | Typical associated features |
|---|---|
| **True organomegaly** | |
| Hepatomegaly | Hepatoblastoma, leukaemia, lymphoma, metabolic disease, hepatitis, EBV, heart failure, haemoglobinopathies, cystic fibrosis |
| Enlarged kidney | Wilms' tumour, neuroblastoma, polycystic kidney |
| Splenomegaly | Lymphoma, leukaemia, EBV, haemoglobinopathies, portal hypertension |
| Testis | Cyst, tumour, torsion |
| **Apparent organomegaly** | |
| Palpable liver, normal size | Hyperexpansion of lungs, pushing liver down |
| Suprapubic mass | Full bladder, pregnancy |
| Scrotal enlargement | Hernia, hydrocoele |
| **Other masses** | |
| Smooth pelvic mass | Ovarian cyst |
| Soft left iliac fossa mass | Stool |
| Epigastric olive-shaped mass | Pyloric stenosis |
| Tender iliac fossa mass | Psoas abscess |
| Reducible protrusion | Hernias |
| EBV – Epstein-Barr Virus, the cause of infectious mononucleosis. | |

**Table 8.5** Causes of abdominal masses

## 8.3 Examination of the abdomen

The paediatric abdominal examination follows the same basic format as in adults. However, because a child may not be compliant, you often have to restructure the order and use windows of opportunity for palpation.

A sequence for examining the abdomen is:
- general inspection
- hands
- pulses and blood pressure
- head and neck

- chest
- abdomen
- investigations

## General inspection
### Exposure

Most children can be positioned as with an adult, lying flat on a bed and undressed down to their underwear. Some children prefer to be examined on their parent's lap: compliance is easier, but clinical signs are often harder to interpret. Watch the child closely during exposure. Valuable clues can be gained from how easily a child climbs onto the bed, sits up or takes off their top.

### General assessment

First, stand back and inspect the child's overall appearance, in particular assessing:
- clinical state
- hydration status
- dysmorphia
- growth (height and weight)
- colour
- scars (**Figure 8.2**)
- implants for feeding (**Figure 8.3**)

### Hands

Signs of abdominal disease in the hands include:
- clubbing – seen in inflammatory bowel disease and coeliac disease
- leukonychia (pale, white nails) – seen in anaemia
- koilonychia (spoon-shaped nails) – seen in iron deficiency
- pallor of the palmar creases – seen in anaemia

### Pulses and BP

- Check the peripheral pulse. An elevated pulse can be a sign of sepsis, dehydration or pain
- BP may be low in sepsis or severe dehydration. It rises in renal disease or if the child is in pain

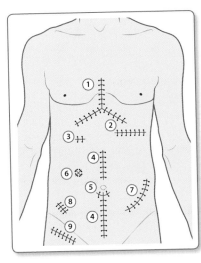

**Figure 8.2** Scars indicating previous abdominal surgery. ① Liver transplant, ② congenital diaphragmatic hernia repair or splenectomy, ③ pyloric stenosis repair, ④ laparotomy, ⑤ umbilical hernia repair, ⑥ drain or laparoscopy, ⑦ renal transplant, ⑧ appendectomy, ⑨ inguinal hernia repair.

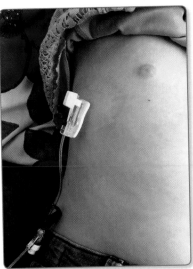

**Figure 8.3** A central line may be used for regular blood tests or to administer parenteral nutrition. This indwelling central venous catheter has been 'accessed' with a 90-degree access needle (Huber).

## Head and neck
### Eyes

Signs in the eyes can suggest the presence of abdominal disease, for example if there is:

- jaundice – in liver disease or haemolysis
- periorbital oedema – in nephrotic syndrome
- xanthelasma – abnormal lipid deposits around the eyes in children with an abnormal lipid profile
- pallor of the conjunctivae – a sign of anaemia
- Kayser–Fleischer rings – blue–green rings of copper deposit around the iris that are seen in Wilson's disease

### Mouth

Inspect for anatomical abnormalities (e.g. cleft lip) and poor dentition, both of which affect the child's ability to feed.
  Specific abnormalities in the mouth include:

- brown perioral pigmentation – in Peutz–Jegher syndrome (hereditary intestinal polyposis syndrome)
- atrophic glossitis – deficiency of iron, vitamin $B_{12}$ and folate
- aphthous ulcers – associated with Crohn's disease
- sweet-smelling breath – diabetic ketoacidosis or liver failure (hepatic fetor)

### Neck

Feel for lymphadenopathy in the cervical and axiliary areas. Marked weight loss with abdominal pain and lymphadenopathy should be investigated for abdominal tuberculosis or lymphoma.

### Chest

Most signs of abdominal disease in the chest are detected by inspection. Look for:

- gynaecomastia – is often benign during puberty but is, rarely, a sign of chronic liver disease in boys
- spider naevi – blanching blood vessels; more than five spider naevi above the nipple line suggests chronic liver disease
- centripetal obesity – fat deposition over the chest and back occurs in Cushing's syndrome and with corticosteroid use

Chest auscultation should be performed because a lower lobe pneumonia often presents with abdominal pain.

## Abdomen

Abdominal examination follows the classic sequence of:

- inspection
- palpation
- percussion
- auscultation

### Inspection

Note whether there is distension. Toddlers often have a protuberant abdomen, and this must be differentiated from an abnormally distended abdomen, which should be measured. Umbilical hernias (**Figure 8.4**) are common in newborns and, if reducible, often spontaneously resolve over the first 2 years of life.

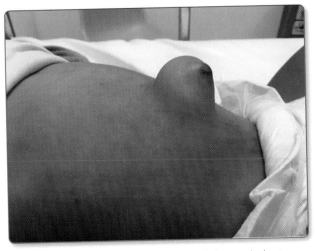

**Figure 8.4** An umbilical hernia. This is easily reducible, but pops back out on coughing.

## Clinical insight

It is a common mistake to look at the abdomen when you are palpating. Always look at the child's face: they may grimace rather than declare pain verbally.

Ask the child to 'suck in the tummy' as far as possible, then to 'push it out as far as possible', and then to cough. If the child cannot do these things, you must consider peritonitis.

Inspect the abdomen, including the flanks, for scars suggestive of previous surgery (see **Figure 8.2**). Note stomas or enteral feeding tubes (see **Table 8.6**).

### Palpation

Ask the child to point with one finger to where the pain is worst. Make sure your hands are warm and gently feel the abdomen. Start at the point furthest away from the pain, and always look at the child's face for signs of discomfort or pain.

Feel all areas of the abdomen, initially superficially and then deeper. Note the precise location of:
- tenderness
- masses

Take time to establish whether masses are:
- reducible – ask the child to cough; a hernia that has been reduced before the cough will re-form
- transilluminant – a torch light shone through the mass will illuminate the whole of the mass if it contains clear fluid; this helps to detect infantile hydrocoeles
- pulsatile – as with some vascular masses, e.g. arteriovenous malformations
- resonant – solid or fluid-filled masses are dull to percussion, whereas a gas-filled mass (e.g. a hernia) is resonant
- auscultatable – bowel sounds may be heard in a hernia, and a bruit may be heard over vascular masses
- fluctuant – a cystic lesion may be an abscess that can be drained
- tender – this is suggestive of local infection or inflammation and not just enlargement per se

Feel formally for a liver and spleen. With the hand in the right iliac fossa, ask the child to breathe in and out. Gently advance

| Device | Anatomical course | Appearance | Function |
|---|---|---|---|
| Nasogastric tube | Through nostril into stomach | Plastic tube entering nostril | Temporary bolus feeding and medication administration |
| Nasojejunal tube | Through nostril, stomach and duodenum into jejunum | Plastic tube entering nostril | Non-surgical continuous feeding via pump, and drug administration, bypassing stomach |
| PEG button | Through skin of epigastrium/ hypochondrium into stomach | Valve-like plastic button in abdominal wall | Bolus feeding and medication administration |
| PEJ tube | Through skin of epigastrium/ hypochondrium, stomach, and duodenum into jejunum | Simple tube, often with a triangular clip, through abdominal wall | Continuous feeding via pump, and drug administration, bypassing stomach |
| PEG-J tube | Through skin of epigastrium/ hypochondrium with one exit port in stomach, and a tube running through duodenum into jejunum | Double lumen tube through valve-like plastic button in abdominal wall, labelled 'G' and 'J' respectively | Options of continuous feeding using pump via J-tube (e.g. at night) and bolus feeding/ drug administration via gastric tube (e.g. during day) |

G, gastrostomy; J, jejunostomy; PE, percutaneous endoscopic

**Table 8.6** Implants for feeding seen in paediatric patients

the tips of your index and middle fingers, holding them fairly superficially, up toward the costal margin. In a child up to 1 year of age, it is normal to be able to feel approximately 1 cm of liver.

To feel for the spleen, use the same technique as for the liver, moving the fingers from the right iliac fossa to the left hypochondrium.

Feel for enlarged kidneys using ballottement. Place one hand on the child's back at the costophrenic angle. Place the other hand on the anterior of the abdomen in the same region. Then, using the hand on the back, attempt to lift the kidney to touch the other hand. A palpable kidney is generally enlarged.

The differential diagnosis of abdominal organomegaly is summarised in **Table 8.5**.

## Percussion

Percuss masses to elicit whether they contain gas (the percussion note will be resonant) or are solid (the percussion note will be dull).

Assess for shifting dullness, which indicates ascites (**Figure 8.5**). With the child lying supine, ascitic fluid should fall to the flanks. Because the gas-containing bowel floats on the fluid, the central abdomen will be resonant to percussion, and the flanks will be dull. Next ask the child to turn on to the left side. Wait for a minute and then percuss again over the central area. If this is now dull to percussion, the fluid has shifted to the new position and ascites is present.

## Auscultation

Listen for bowel sounds, noting their presence and quality. High-pitched, tinkling, overactive sounds indicate distal

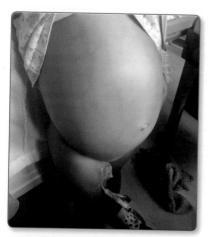

**Figure 8.5** Abdominal distention due to ascites. Fluid is retained in the abdomen owing to low serum albumin in liver disease and nephrotic syndrome.

obstruction. Listen for 60 seconds; absent bowel sounds suggest an ileus.

Listen over masses and over the kidneys for bruits (soft murmurs caused by turbulent blood flow through abnormal blood vessels).

## Further examination

To complete the examination of the abdominal system:

- look at the groins for inguinal hernias
- if indicated by localised pain, examine the external genitalia, particularly to rule out testicular torsion
- look at the child's back to rule out spina bifida as a cause of constipation
- look for rashes, particularly nappy rash (see page 240) and erythema nodosum (see page 253)

## Investigations

After the examination, a number of investigations should be considered, depending on the presenting symptoms. Investigations include:

- dipstick urine test
- urine culture
- stool culture
- blood pressure
- abdominal ultrasound
- contrast study
- oesophageal pH study

Abdominal radiographs are of limited use in children with diarrhoea or vomiting because, unlike the chest, the internal viscera are not visualised on a radiograph. Causes of obstruction, such as intussusception and pyloric stenosis are best seen on ultrasound.

## Clinical insight

In children, rectal examination should be avoided where possible. It should only be carried out by the doctor whose management plan it will alter, for example a surgeon deciding whether to perform a rectal biopsy for Hirschprung's disease.

## 8.4 Examination summary

A summary of the abdominal examination is given in **Table 8.7**.

| Component | Assessment/key findings |
|---|---|
| General inspection | Is the child well or unwell? Is the child in pain? Height and weight |
| Around the bed | Specialist feeds, vomit bowls |
| Hands | Clubbing, nails, palmar erythema |
| Face | Eyes, tongue, dentition, breath, mouth ulcers |
| Chest | Gynaecomastia, obesity |
| Abdomen | Scars, masses, distension, fluid, stomas |
| Other | Groins, back, legs |
| Investigations | Urine dipstick, urine microscopy, stool virology, culture and biochemistry |
| Have you ruled out... ? | Intra-abdominal masses, peritonitis, appendicitis, severe dehydration, tuberculosis, lymphoma |

**Table 8.7** Summary of the paediatric abdominal examination

# The nervous system

Abnormalities of brain, spine and neuromuscular function present with probably the widest variety of symptoms in paediatric medicine. Although neurological problems present as common symptoms such as headache, squint, weakness or seizures, such symptoms do not often indicate underlying brain or spine pathology. Headaches, for example, are usually idiopathic, and febrile convulsions are far more common than epilepsy.

The neurological examination should therefore be thought of in two ways. First, it is a screening tool to rule out a rare neurological cause of common symptoms. Second, it is a way of identifying the precise location of a pathology.

## Approaching the examination

Neurological examination overlaps significantly with developmental examination (see **Chapter 5**). The brain and spine are plastic, evolving, entities in children, so even establishing 'normal' levels of function can prove a challenge. The key is to develop skills by seeing and examining as many children as possible, for example identifying what is a normal broad-based gait in a 14-month-old who is learning to walk, and comparing it with the similar posture of a 4-year-old with ataxia.

It takes repeated practice to be able to elicit solid clinical signs, such as reflexes and squints, especially in younger children who struggle to comply with a formal examination. Ingenuity is required to assess movement, strength, tone and reflexes. It is often necessary to invent games on the spur of the moment, use a variety of means of distraction (see **Chapter 3**) or employ the help of a play therapist.

# 9.1 Clinical scenarios

## Acute onset of ataxia

A 5-year-old girl presents to the emergency department with sudden-onset ataxia that has been rapidly progressing for the past 48 hours: she now cannot walk unaided. She was previously fit and well, other than a recent mild case of chickenpox. There has been no head injury, and no complaints of recent headaches, visual disturbance or hearing loss.

She is finding it difficult to eat by herself, because her hands seem to be shaking. She is alert, otherwise happy and not on medication.

## Differential diagnosis

This includes:

- cerebellitis
- stroke
- posterior fossa tumour
- Friedreich's ataxia
- gluten ataxia
- Guillain–Barré syndrome
- encephalitis/encephalopathy
- drug toxicity
- Wilson's disease

## Further information

While the child is sitting, her trunk is unsteady and she is swaying from side to side. Her face appears normal, with no weakness or asymmetry, although there is some horizontal nystagmus and her speech is unclear. A few healing chickenpox lesions are present on the face and trunk.

There are normal power, tone and tendon reflexes, but a marked tremor when the child tries to touch her nose with her fingers. Lower limb examination appears normal, with normal ankle and knee reflexes.

## Conclusion

This girl has acute ataxia, and the signs point to a cerebellar lesion. There is no history of fever, headaches or reduced conscious level, which rules out encephalitis and acute disseminated encephalomyelitis. There has not been no exposure to drugs. Peripheral reflexes and lower limb power are normal, making Guillain–Barré syndrome unlikely. There is no jaundice, and the child is too young to be showing symptoms of Wilson's disease which classically presents in adolescence.

The most likely diagnosis is an acute viral (chickenpox-related) cerebellitis.

## Acute symmetrical lower limb weakness

A 10-year-old boy presents with a 4-day history of increasing weakness of his legs, first noticed when playing football. There has also been worsening lower back pain, and his lower legs and thighs feel weak.

He is normally fit and well. However, about 2 weeks ago he had food poisoning, with some bloody diarrhoea, after a family holiday in Egypt. This resolved with antibiotics prescribed by the GP. The child is fully immunised.

### Differential diagnosis

The differential diagnosis for lower limb weakness includes:
- encephalitis/encephalomyelitis
- Guillain–Barré syndrome
- spinal tumour
- anterior horn diseases
- myositis
- myelitis
- peripheral neuropathy
- botulism
- polio

### Further information

The child is alert and interacting normally, and has no obvious facial weakness. Vital signs, including temperature, are normal. He is able to walk very slowly, and he complains of weakness and pain in his lower back as he walks.

There is no tingling of his legs. Urinary output is good, although there is mild constipation. There are no other symptoms, for example headaches, fevers, cough or abdominal pain.

There are no abnormal findings on examination of the arms. The legs show no evidence of muscle wasting, fasciculation or tenderness on palpation. There is significant weakness and reduced muscle tone of all muscle groups from hip to toes. The knee and ankle reflexes are reduced. Sensation seems normal. Examination of the lower back reveals no overlying swelling and no localised tenderness.

### Conclusion

There is hypotonia and hyporeflexia, so this is a peripheral neuropathy. Guillain–Barré syndrome is the most common cause of acute flaccid paralysis and has a strong association with *Campylobacter* infection; this could have been the cause of the bloody diarrhoea.

The lack of sphincter disturbance makes transverse myelitis unlikely, but this should be excluded with MRI and lumbar puncture (see page 158).

Immunisation and symmetrical symptoms make polio unlikely. Positive neurological abnormality and lack of tenderness rule out myositis. Acute myasthenia is rare, and there is no facial or upper limb abnormality to suggest such an autoimmune pathology.

## 9.2 Common presentations

Key presentations of neurological conditions in children include:
- a 'lazy' eye
- headache
- seizures
- weakness
- hypotonia
- hypertonia
- ataxia
- altered sensation with weakness

### A 'lazy' eye

One eye, the 'lazy' eye, is misaligned with the direction in which the child is looking. This can lead to permanent visual impairment (amblyopia) as the brain stops perceiving the image received from the misaligned eye. When this has a neuromuscular cause, it is termed strabismus.

## Strabismus (squint)

The degree of squinting ranges from a squint that is obvious to others to one that is detectable only using a cover test (see page 149).

The differential diagnosis is as follows:

- Non-paralytic strabismus (common) – this is commonly found in children who have refractive errors, the squint helping them accommodate for these
- Paralytic strabismus (rare) – a cranial nerve palsy affecting the extraocular muscles. For example a VIth nerve (abducens nerve) palsy causes a fixed convergent squint; this can occur with raised intracranial pressure caused by an intracranial tumour
- Pseudosquint (common) – the eyes are perfectly aligned but a unilateral epicanthic fold (see **Chapter 14**) causes the pupil of one eye to appear to lie more medially than the other

*Clinical features*  The typical appearance of a squint is a misalignment of the eyes, so they appear to focus in slightly different directions. In the common non-paralytic type, both eyes move in all directions when tested; in the rare paralytic type, one eye will not move in one or more directions.

## Headache

Headache is one of the most common presentations in school age children and adolescents. It is challenging to establish the difference between a benign and a serious cause. Causes of headache include:

- tension headache
- migraine
- intracranial tumour

### Tension headache

*Clinical features*  Tension headaches are usually frontal or bilateral, and may be associated with aching neck muscles. They are much more common than migraines, and there are no associated features such as vomiting or visual disturbances. A tension

## Clinical insight

Vision should be checked in children suffering from tension headaches – they may simply need corrective spectacles.

headache is frequently associated with everyday triggers, such as long periods spent in front of a bright screen, lack of adequate hydration, prolonged visual concentration or stress.

### Migraine

*Clinical features* In some patients, migraines begin with an aura (abnormal sensations of taste or vision). The headaches are usually frontal or unilateral, and may be pulsating in nature. Associated symptoms include nausea, vomiting and photophobia. The headache may last for hours or days.

## Clinical insight

Be careful to distinguish neck pain from 'neck stiffness'. Agonising headache, exacerbated when the meninges stretch on neck movement, is a sign of meningitis. Many people refer to 'neck stiffness' despite a full range of movement in the neck muscles with some pain.

If there are focal neurological symptoms, such as limb weakness, MRI of the brain, with magnetic resonance angiography (MRA) of cerebral blood vessels, are required to exclude an arteriovenous malformation.

### Intracranial tumour

Tumours inside the skull (space-occupying lesions) cause mass effects (compression of the brain) and raised intracranial pressure. Brain tumours are the most common solid malignancy of children.

## Clinical insight

Vomiting in the mornings is a symptom of brain tumour or pregnancy. The standard pregnancy test measures β-human chorionic gonadotropin, which may be raised in intracranial germinomas. Therefore always remember to organise MRI of the brain if there is a positive pregnancy test but a negative pelvic ultrasound result.

*Clinical features* The symptoms of raised intracranial pressures are headaches, nausea and vomiting, predominantly in the morning, that ease through the day. There may be visual disturbance and papilloedema. Focal neurological signs arise from compression of nearby areas of the brain, whose function will be disrupted. Seizures may also occur.

## Seizures

Seizures are the result of a chaotic discharge of electricity in the brain. They are either generalised (affecting the whole body) or focal (affecting one part of the body).

**Differential diagnosis**  Seizures may be the presentation of:
- febrile convulsion
- epilepsy
- intracranial infection (meningitis, encephalitis or abscess)
- intracranial mass (tumour or neurofibroma)
- brain injury (acute or chronic)
- hypoglycaemia
- hyponatraemia

> ### Clinical insight
> Hypoglycaemia is a cause of seizures. A normal blood sugar test in children with seizures rules this out.

### Febrile convulsion

A febrile convulsion is a seizure that occurs during a period of pyrexia. The cause is unknown, but there is often a family history of febrile convulsions. They can be recurrent but are not a form of epilepsy. The condition is benign and requires no treatment.

*Clinical features*  Febrile convulsions occur between 6 months and 6 years of age. They are usually brief (<5 minutes) and generalised (the child loses consciousness and shakes all four limbs). They can also be followed by a postictal phase of drowsiness. These features help to differentiate a febrile convulsion from rigors, in which a febrile child shivers but does not lose consciousness.

### Epilepsy

Epilepsy is defined as recurrent non-febrile seizures. It can follow an insult to the brain (e.g. cerebral palsy), relate to a cortical malformation or have no clear cause.

*Clinical features*  Seizures are focal or generalised. Focal seizures affect one area of the body; there may be lip smacking, a repeated spasm of the hand or a brief moment of vacant staring (an absence seizure).

Generalised seizures present as collapse and uncontrollable shaking. There may also be tongue biting or urinary incontinence.

## Weakness

Weakness can be caused by any insult to the central nervous system (CNS), the peripheral nerve or the muscle (**Figure 9.1**). When considering the differential diagnosis (**Table 9.1**), establish whether:

- affected areas are floppy (hypotonia) or stiff (hypertonia)
- weakness is acute or chronic
- the problem is generalised or isolated to one area

## Hypotonia

Hypotonia is decreased tone (floppiness). Decreased tone may be associated with weakness, and the differential diagnoses of the two overlap.

**Differential diagnosis** There are many possible causes of hypotonia (**Table 9.1**). Differential diagnoses include:

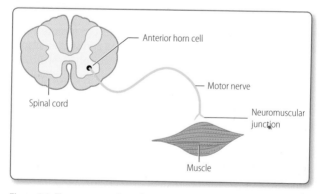

**Figure 9.1** The neuromuscular pathway.

|  | Hypertonia | Hypotonia | Normal tone |
|---|---|---|---|
| Generalised causes | Hypocalcaemia (tetany) | Down's syndrome Prader–Willi syndrome Hypothyroidism Inborn errors of metabolism | Hypothyroidism Depression Functional disorders |
| Acute infective causes | Meningitis Encephalitis Abscess Tetanus | Polio Botulism | Acute myositis Dermatomyositis |
| Acute non-infective causes | Late stroke Intracranial lesion | Early stroke Guillain–Barré syndrome Neuromuscular blockers* |  |
| Chronic causes | Cerebral palsy Intracranial lesion | Spinal muscular atrophy Peripheral neuropathy Myasthenia gravis | Muscular dystrophy |
| Acute or chronic causes | Demyelination Head trauma | Nerve root compression Body trauma | Musculoskeletal diagnoses |

*Drugs including acetylcholine esterase inhibitors, suxamethonium and curare derivatives such as atracurium.

Table 9.1 Key causes of weakness with neurological signs

- an inherited syndrome, e.g. Down's syndrome (see page 287)
- a genetic abnormality, e.g. spinal muscular atrophy
- infection (polio or botulism)
- stroke

Spinal muscular atrophy
Spinal muscular atrophy is a recessively inherited condition (see Chapter 14) that causes degeneration of neurones in the anterior spinal cord.

*Clinical features*  Children present in the neonatal period with hypotonia, or at 6–9 months when they miss key motor milestones (see **Chapter 5**) such as sitting. There is generalised floppiness with soft to absent reflexes and tongue fasciculation. The condition deteriorates with time, with the proximal muscles of the arms and legs being most rapidly affected. Children with an *SMN1* gene mutation can be treated with nusinersen, which has only recently been approved in the UK, EU and USA.

## Poliomyelitis

Poliovirus infection affects the anterior horn cells of the spinal cord.

*Clinical features*  Poliovirus infection is initially asymptomatic or produces a mild flu-like illness or gastroenteritis. Lower motor neurone signs – weakness, hypotonia and absent reflexes – then develop. The virus does not infect every anterior horn cell so signs are asymmetric and more commonly unilateral than bilateral.

## Botulism

Botulism is caused by a toxin produced by *Clostridium botulinum*, a bacterium that is found in uncooked meat. The toxin blocks the neuromuscular junctions.

*Clinical features*  Initial *Clostridium* infection may produce a gastroenteritis, but the classic clinical feature is of a rapidly progressing, full-body flaccid paralysis. Affected children may require mechanical ventilation.

## Stroke

A stroke occurs when the arterial blood supply to an area of cerebral cortex is suddenly stopped, by bleeding or thrombosis. This results in the death of neurones that depend on the affected artery.

Unlike in adults, atherosclerotic thrombosis is rare in children. The aetiology is more commonly:

- an underlying condition causing a prothrombotic state (e.g. malignancy)

- vascular abnormality (e.g. narrowing of the artery after chickenpox)
- vessel occlusion from clots of abnormal blood cells (e.g. sickle cell disease)

*Clinical features*  There is sudden-onset unilateral hypotonia, and often difficulty with speech production. This gradually evolves into hypertonia: a stiff contracted limb with brisk reflexes (see Hypertonia section below). Newborn babies may have seizures following a stroke.

## Hypertonia

Hypertonia is increased tone, also known as spasticity. The affected region (which may be a limb or the trunk) is held stiff, and it is difficult to move it passively. Hypertonia occurs when there is damage to the CNS system (an 'upper motor neurone lesion'), resulting in brisk reflexes and weakness.

**Differential diagnosis**  Causes of hypertonia other than intra-cranial infection include:

- cerebral palsy
- acute disseminated encephalomyelitis
- stroke (see page 154)

### Cerebral palsy

Cerebral palsy is defined as a 'fixed insult to the developing brain'. The common causes are:

- genetic abnormality
- hypoxic–ischaemic brain injury
- prolonged hypoglycaemia
- intraventricular haemorrhage (which may occur in prema-ture neonates)
- infection, e.g. meningitis
- trauma from a head injury

*Clinical features*  The pattern of signs depends on the site of injury and the child's developing abilities. Signs range from mild, for example a hemiplegic gait in an otherwise normal child, to severe, such as disability involving movement, vision, hearing, swallowing and oesophageal motility. Children with severe cerebral palsy are at risk of aspiration and pneumonia as well as seizure disorders.

## Acute disseminated encephalomyelitis

Acute disseminated encephalomyelitis (ADEM) is an immune-mediated destruction of the myelin sheath of the neurones. It usually follows a viral illness and is particularly associated with measles.

*Clinical features*  Presentation is usually 2–3 weeks after a viral infection with weakness and features of encephalopathy (decreased consciousness and seizures). It is treated with corticosteroids. A small proportion of children go on to develop multiple sclerosis, but the first presentation of multiple sclerosis does not usually include the encephalopathy characteristic of ADEM.

## Ataxia

Damage to, or inflammation of, the cerebellum can cause widespread deficits in coordination. Pathologies that cause ataxia are detailed in **Table 9.2**.

| Cause | Examples |
|---|---|
| Immunological | Chickenpox (varicella zoster virus) <br> Gluten ataxia* |
| Genetic | Ataxia telangiectasia <br> Friedreich's ataxia |
| Compression | Posterior fossa tumour <br> Arnold–Chiari malformation |
| Stroke | Vertebral artery stroke |
| Drugs | Antiepileptics <br> Alcohol <br> Benzodiazepines <br> Ketamine |
| Error of copper metabolism | Wilson's disease |
| *Damage to cerebellar neurones from cross-reaction with antigliadin antibodies. | |

**Table 9.2** Causes of ataxia

*Clinical features*  The child walks unsteadily with a broad-based gait. There may be rapid beating eye movements at rest (nystagmus) or on lateral gaze. Speech may be slurred (dysarthria). There is impaired reaching for objects, with overreaching and an intention tremor.

## Clinical insight

Ataxia-like symptoms are seen in patients with sensory neuropathies – so-called 'sensory ataxia'. Poor proprioceptive feedback makes it difficult for the cerebellum to coordinate movement. Always consider a sensory problem in patients with coordination defects but normal tone.

The child may be very wobbly at rest (titubation). In toddlers, ask what their baseline motor function and development is for comparison (see **Chapter 5**).

## Altered sensation with weakness

Numbness and tingling are very common symptoms – everyone has had 'pins and needles' from lying on a limb awkwardly. However, these symptoms should be very short-lived. Continuing paraesthesia is often a sign of significant pathology, particularly if combined with weakness or coordination difficulties. Establish whether there is a dermatomal level above which there is a normal examination but below which there is abnormal sensation. This is a prime indicator of a spinal pathology.

**Differential diagnosis**  Numbness or tingling with weakness can be symptomatic of:

- spinal tumour
- transverse myelitis
- Guillain–Barré syndrome
- multiple sclerosis
- lead poisoning

### Spinal tumour

Spinal tumours are relatively rare compared with brain tumours, comprising 5% of all CNS tumours. The most common types are astrocytomas, dermoid and epidermoid tumours, and neuroblastomas. Some bone tumours present in the spine.

## Clinical insight

Back pain is not a common presentation in children. Most childhood back pain is symptomatic of a significant pathology and requires full examination and MRI.

*Clinical features* Spinal tumours commonly present as a mixture of numbness and weakness below a specific dermatomal level. There is often focal back pain, which is exquisitely tender over the tumour. There may be dysfunction of the bowel or bladder, such as secondary nocturnal enuresis (bedwetting; see page 274), and this can be the primary presenting symptom.

### Transverse myelitis

This is inflammatory demyelination across the width of the spinal cord at a specific level. It has many causes, most of which are infective. These include HIV, Epstein–Barr virus, cytomegalovirus, herpes simplex virus, Zika virus, *Campylobacter* diarrhoea, Lyme disease (see page 247) and *Mycoplasma* infection. It also presents as part of multiple sclerosis (see page 159).

*Clinical features* Transverse myelitis has a clear set of diagnostic and exclusion criteria, listed in **Table 9.3**.

| Positive criteria | Exclusion criteria |
|---|---|
| Spinal motor or sensory dysfunction | Recent spinal radiotherapy |
| Bilateral symptoms (not necessarily symmetrical) | Presence of tumour or arteriovenous malformation |
| Clear sensory level | Optic neuritis |
| Signs of inflammation on lumbar puncture or MRI | Multiple sclerosis on lumbar puncture or MRI |
| Peak symptoms no earlier than 4 hours | Evidence of connective tissue disease |
| Peak symptoms no later than 21 days | Evidence of local or systemic infection |

**Table 9.3** Transverse Myelitis Consortium Working Group Diagnostic Criteria (2002)

## Guillain–Barré syndrome

Guillain–Barré syndrome is an acute inflammatory polyneuropathy of the peripheral nerves. It is a post-infective pathology, most commonly triggered by *Streptococcus, Pneumococcus* and *Campylobacter* spp.. *Mycoplasma* is a much rarer cause. Several viruses cause Guillain–Barré syndrome, including Epstein–Barr, varicella zoster, influenza and Zika viruses.

*Clinical features*   After a prodromal illness, the child develops altered sensation, usually starting at the tips of the fingers and toes. This ascends rapidly over a few hours to a few days. The sensory symptoms can include neuropathic pain. Other symptoms include weakness, hypotonia and reduced reflexes. Around 15% of children require intubation and ventilation, as the paralysis reaches the muscles of respiration.

The cerebrospinal fluid shows a normal white blood cell count but elevated protein. MRI shows enhancement of the spinal nerve roots in 95% of cases. Nerve conduction studies show the slowed activity of demyelination.

## Multiple sclerosis

Multiple sclerosis is an idiopathic demyelinating condition of the CNS. It affects the brain, spine and optic nerves. There is a relapsing and remitting clinical course, most commonly with a progressive deterioration (each remission does not bring the patient back to the premorbid baseline). It is rare in children.

*Clinical features*   Children with multiple sclerosis present with almost any combination of neurological symptoms, so diagnosis is challenging. One clue is that symptoms are often worse in hot environments (Uhthoff's sign). Symptoms include hypertonia, hyperreflexia, weakness and altered sensation in isolated or multiple areas. Blurring of vision and problems with red-spectrum colour vision are characteristic of optic neuritis, which occurs in around a quarter of patients. An electric shock on tilting the head forward (the barber's chair phenomenon) is common. Diagnosis is by MRI and confirmation of oligoclonal bands in the cerebrospinal fluid.

### Lead poisoning

Lead poisoning has become much less common in developed countries as lead is no longer used in pipes and paints. The most common cause is chronic unwitting ingestion of contaminated substances; acute high-dose consumption is much less common.

*Clinical features*   The classic presentation is with tingling in the arms and legs against the background of chronic abdominal pain. There are often headaches, constipation, anaemia and irritability. There is usually a history of pica (see page 273) that explains the regular ingestion of paint or metal.

## 9.3 Examination of the nervous system

The neurological examination is a multistage examination of all aspects of sensation, movement and higher function. It should be performed in conjunction with a developmental assessment (see **Chapter 5**) and a behavioural assessment (see **Chapter 13**) to provide as many clues as possible to guide diagnosis and management.

A suggested sequence for the neurological examination is:
- general assessment
- mobility
- cranial nerves
- limbs
  - tone
  - power and muscle function
  - tendon reflexes
  - sensation
- cerebellar examination
- primitive and protective reflexes (in infants)

### Exposure

To perform the examination properly, the child should be undressed to their underwear. It is easy to miss neurocutaneous markers, fasciculations and gait abnormalities in a fully clothed child.

## General assessment

This should include:
- general appearance
- conscious level
- the skin

## General appearance

Look for obvious clues to underlying neurological disease. Examine for:
- dysmorphia and skull shape (see page 306)
- abnormal posture (see page 195)
- lack of visual alertness, i.e. lack of fixed gaze on objects or faces (see **Chapter 5**)
- height, weight and head circumference (see **Chapter 4**)

Clues to a child's level of neurological function are:
- a wheelchair
- hearing aids
- feeding or gastrostomy tubes
- use of nappies in a school-age child
- splints to support hypertonic legs
- scars from previous craniectomy or tendon releases
- a palpable ventriculoperitoneal shunt under the skin of the occiput and neck – the treatment for hydrocephalus

## Conscious level

The Glasgow Coma Scale (**Table 9.4**) was initially developed for assessing adults with head injuries, but it has been adapted for children. It rates three areas of response, with a total score ranging from 3 to 15. A score <15 is concerning, and intubation and ventilation should be considered if the score is ≤8.

Always ask the parent what the child's baseline function is, and use common sense to adjust your

### Clinical insight

There is a great difference between an 'irritable' child and an 'unsettled' child. 'Irritable' is used in healthcare settings to mean 'distressed and irritable' – the more you do to calm them, the worse they get; this is a sign of meningoencephalitis. 'Unsettled' refers to a child who is 'distressed and settleable' – attempts to mollify the child have some positive effect.

|  | Infants | Children | Score |
|---|---|---|---|
| Eye opening | Open spontaneously | Open spontaneously | 4 |
|  | Open in response to verbal stimuli | Open in response to verbal stimuli | 3 |
|  | Open in response to pain only | Open in response to pain only | 2 |
|  | No response | No response | 1 |
| Verbal response | Coos and babbles | Orientated, appropriate | 5 |
|  | Irritable cries | Confused | 4 |
|  | Cries in response to pain | Inappropriate words | 3 |
|  | Moans in response to pain | Incomprehensible words or non-specific sounds | 2 |
|  | No response | No response | 1 |
| Motor response | Moves spontaneously and purposefully | Obeys commands | 6 |
|  | Withdraws to touch | Localises painful stimulus | 5 |
|  | Withdraws in response to pain | Withdraws in response to pain | 4 |
|  | Responds to pain with decorticate posturing (abnormal flexion) | Responds to pain with flexion | 3 |
|  | Responds to pain with decerebrate posturing (abnormal extension) | Responds to pain with extension | 2 |
|  | No response | No response | 1 |

The three values from each test are considered separately and as a total in assessing conscious level.

Table 9.4 Glasgow Coma Scale in infants and children

assessment using the scale. For example, a shy child may not follow your commands but will follow their parent's.

If you are concerned that a child appears drowsy or unconscious, it is appropriate to firmly rub the child on the sternum with a finger or knuckle. This provides a painful central stimulus that should rouse the child. If a sternal rub is not possible (e.g. because of sternal injury), squeeze the trapezius muscle or apply pressure to the superior orbit.

## Skin (neurocutaneous markers)
Neurocutaneous markers are specific lesions or appearances of
the skin that are associated with neurological disease. Examine
the whole skin, particularly the back and axillae. Some examples
and their associated conditions are listed in **Table 9.5**. Ash leaf
macules are easier to see under a Wood's (blue light) lamp.

## Mobility
The inspection of function overlaps with the developmental
and musculoskeletal examinations (see **Chapters 5** and **10**).
   When assessing mobility, consider:
* limb appearance, tone and muscle bulk
* gait when walking, turning and balance

| Name | Appearance | Associated conditions |
|---|---|---|
| Café-au-lait spot (Coast of California type) | Large, flat, pigmented, smooth perimeter | Neurofibromatosis |
| Café -au-lait spot (Coast of Maine type) | Large, flat, pigmented, ragged perimeter Unilateral | McCune–Albright syndrome* |
| Axillary freckles | Small, flat, pigmented, smooth perimeter in axillae | Neurofibromatosis |
| Port-wine stain | Purple-red birthmark across face | Sturge–Weber syndrome |
| Telangiectasia | Prominent blood vessels, particularly over sclerae and mucosa | Ataxia telangiectasia |
| Shagreen patch | Leathery fibrotic plaque | Tuberous sclerosis |
| Ash leaf macule | Ash leaf shaped, flat area of depigmentation, often over the sacrum | Tuberous sclerosis |
| *McCune-Albright Syndrome – precocious puberty, hyperpituitarism, fibrous dysplasia. | | |

Table 9.5 Neurocutaneous markers, their appearance and associated conditions

## Limb appearance and leg length

Inspect the limbs for:

- posture
- asymmetry
- wasting or hypertrophy
- fasciculations
- scars
- dyskinesias

**Posture**  A hypotonic baby lies in a 'frog-leg' posture with the limbs flat against the cot surface. When they are held, their arms may flop about like a rag doll's. A stiff baby may hold the neck hyperextended and have the knees flexed and the hands in a closed fist (hypertonic). Decorticate posturing is abnormal flexion of the upper limbs, with the legs in extension, caused by lesions to the corticospinal and rubrospinal tract. In decerebrate posturing, all four limbs are held in extension, owing to lesions below the level of the red nucleus in the midbrain and brainstem.

**Limb position**  A hypertonic arm is held tight against the body in tight flexion. A hypertonic leg rests in extension. A lower motor neurone lesion produces a loose arm. For example, in Erb's palsy, the elbow is extended, and the forearm pronated (the 'waiter's tip' posture); this results from a brachial plexus injury caused by the shoulder becoming trapped in the birth canal during birth.

**Asymmetry**  Unilateral neurological disease is sometimes obvious. In polio, for example, there is usually pronounced muscle wasting in one limb.

**Wasting**  Muscle wasting suggests prolonged underuse, and therefore a chronic pathology (**Table 9.1**).

**Hypertrophy**  Muscle hypertrophy in the lower limbs – specifically in the gastrocnemius and soleus muscles – is found in muscular dystrophy. It compensates for the weakness of more proximal muscles.

**Fasciculation** This refers to flickering movements under the skin, caused by individual muscle bundle contractions in the absence of regular stimulation from coordinated motor neurone outputs.

**Scars** Look for scars around the major tendons as a sign of previous tendon release surgery.

**Dyskinesias** These are abnormal movements suggestive of basal ganglia damage:
- athetoid movements are slow and writhing movements
- choreas are involuntary jerky movements

### Assessing gait

Gait abnormalities and their associated pathologies are described in **Table 9.6**.

| Abnormality | Appearance | Associated conditions |
|---|---|---|
| Antalgic | Stance is abnormally brief compared with swing phase on affected side | Musculoskeletal pain |
| Broad based | Staggering, toddling gait, widespread feet. Staggering at rest (titubation) | Cerebellar ataxia |
| Foot drop | Weakness of foot dorsiflexion. Raises leg high to avoid scraping foot on ground | Peripheral motor neuropathy |
| Sweeping | Plantarflexed foot and toes. Hypertonic leg is circumducted during walking | Hemiplegia |
| Scissoring | Hypertonic legs drag when walking and cross the midline owing to stiffness of hip adductors | Diplegia |
| Stamping | High stamping steps without weakness of foot dorsiflexion owing to poor proprioceptive feedback | Sensory neuropathy |
| Waddling | Dropping of the hip girdle on side contralateral to muscle weakness | Proximal muscle weakness |

**Table 9.6** Gait abnormalities and their underlying pathologies

Ask the child if they can walk: a child who is in a wheelchair may still be able to walk a few steps with help.

If the child can walk, ask them to walk away from you and observe the gait from behind. Then ask them to stop, turn around and walk back. A balance problem may become obvious when the child is turning.

A child who is old enough should be asked to heel–toe walk, which assesses balance and coordination.

## Cranial nerve (CN) examination

In fully cooperative older children, the approach to cranial nerve examination is the same as is used as for adults. In younger children, a more pragmatic approach, involving observation during play and distraction, is required.

The nerves can be tested in a roughly numerical order by assessing:

- smell
- vision
- eye movements
- face
- hearing and balance
- neck movements
- the oropharynx

### Smell – CN I (olfactory nerve)

Ask the child if he or she has noticed a change in the sense of smell. This may be formally tested using standard odours, but it is not normally tested in routine practice.

### Vision – CN II (optic nerve)

A full visual assessment can be challenging in young children who cannot follow instructions or identify letters of the alphabet. The following need to be assessed:

- responsiveness
- visual fields
- acuity
- light reflexes
- fundoscopy

**Clinical insight**

Do not use flashing or noisy toys to judge visual fields. Children who are blind are able to hear and turn towards a rattle.

**Responsiveness** Does the child look towards objects and faces? Young infants should be able to fix and follow by 6–8 weeks of age (see **Chapter 5**).

**Visual fields** Distract the child with an object in the central field of vision. For older children, this can be your nose, but in younger children a toy is best. Then move a more interesting object into the peripheral fields of vision to ascertain whether the child moves the gaze towards this second object.

**Visual acuity** Children >4 years of age should be able to use a standard Snellen chart. Special Snellen charts are available with pictograms rather than letters, for younger children and those who cannot read. Cover each of the child's eyes in turn to test their vision separately.

**Red reflex** Look for the red reflex as you would in a newborn examination (see **Chapter 2**). From a distance, shine an ophthalmoscope into each eye and look for the red reflection of the retina. A white reflex is very concerning as it suggests serious retinal disease, such as retinoblastoma (page 21).

**Pupillary reflex** Check the pupils for responses to light, including relative afferent pupillary defects.

When a light is shone into only one pupil, both pupils constrict via the direct and consensual light reflexes. When a light is swung from eye to eye, the pupil into which the light is being shone should constrict, and the other pupil should also momentarily constrict before dilating.

With a relative afferent pupillary defect, neither pupil constricts when a light is shone into the affected eye. When the light is shone into the unaffected eye, however, both pupils do constrict.

**Fundoscopy** This is challenging in children of all ages. If optic nerve damage or retinopathy of prematurity is being considered, it is best practice to arrange for an

## Clinical insight

Children sometimes compensate for the diplopia caused by a squint by tilting their head. A child with a permanently tilted head may have a cranial nerve palsy rather than torticollis.

ophthalmologist to review the optic discs after the pupils have been dilated using a mydriatic agent.

## Eye movements – CN III, IV and VI (oculomotor, trochlear and abducens)

Re-examine the pupils: a CN III palsy causes a fixed dilated pupil with ptosis.

Next, examine the eye movements. Older children can hold their head still and follow your finger with their eyes, but younger children may have to be held by their parent while their peripheral vision is engaged with a toy or bubbles. **Table 9.7** details abnormal eye movements and their aetiologies.

It can be difficult to determine whether a squint is caused by a cranial nerve palsy (paralytic squint) or weakness of the muscle (non-paralytic squint), or is not a true squint (pseudosquint). The cover test (**Figure 9.2**) will help distinguish these.

|  | Appearance | Reason |
|---|---|---|
| CN III palsy | Fixed lateral gaze<br>Ptosis<br>Fixed dilated pupil | Paralysis of all eye muscles except lateral rectus<br>Paralysis of levator palpebrae superioris<br>Paralysis of parasympathetic fibres |
| CN IV palsy | Tilted head | Paralysis of superior oblique* |
| CN VI palsy | New failure of lateral gaze | Paralysis of lateral rectus |
| Duane syndrome | Congenital failure of lateral gaze | Miswiring of CN VI into the wrong muscles |
| Pseudosquint | Apparent strabismus, both eyes normal on cover test | Asymmetrical epicanthic folds |
| Non-paralytic squint | Apparent strabismus, lazy eye normalises during cover test | Asymmetrical weakness of eye muscles |
| * The normal action of superior oblique is the internal rotation and depression of the adducted eye ('intorsion') | | |

**Table 9.7** Eye movement defects

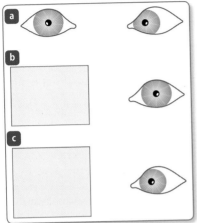

**Figure 9.2** The cover test. (a) A strabismus of the left eye is investigated by covering the right. (b) A non-paralytic squint corrects. (c) A paralytic squint remains misaligned.

For the cover test, sit immediately in front of the child and get the child to fix on an object. Cover the child's good eye while watching the squinting eye. If the squinting eye was not correctly aligned, it should move into the correct visual axis if weak eye muscles do still have a nerve supply (non-paralytic squint). If the eye remains misaligned, the eye muscles have no nerve supply and there is a paralytic squint.

### The face – CN V and VII (trigeminal and facial)

In older children, CN V is tested by asking them to report when their face is gently brushed with cotton wool over the facial dermatomes (**Figure 9.3**). Younger children cannot do this, but you can ask the parents whether there are problems with opening the jaw or chewing as a small motor portion of CN V innervates muscles in the jaw.

> ### Clinical insight
>
> Lyme disease is a cause of facial nerve palsy and needs to be urgently ruled out by serological testing. The facial nerve palsy of Lyme disease resolves spontaneously, falsely reassuring the clinician, and more serious complications only manifest many weeks later.

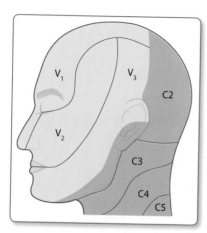

**Figure 9.3** Facial dermatomes. V: trigeminal nerve roots - V₁, ophthalmic nerve; V₂, maxillary nerve; V₃, mandibular nerve. C: cervical spinal nerve roots.

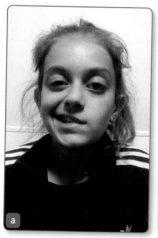 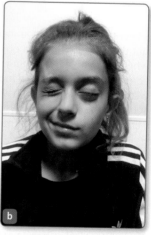

**Figure 9.4** A girl with Bell's palsy. Note that the right eye can be closed more tightly than the left. This is a particular problem when sleeping because the eyes will become very dry.

CN VII is an easily assessed cranial nerve because weakness (Bell's palsy) becomes apparent when the child is asked to smile (**Figure 9.4**). Asking the child to copy 'funny faces' (**Figure 9.5**) is

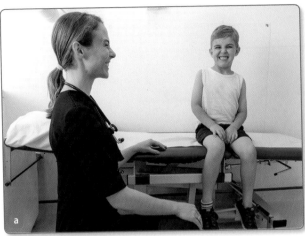

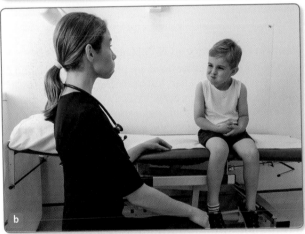

**Figure 9.5** Pulling silly faces tests muscles such as buccinator and levator labii.
*Continues on next page*

a good way of making the examination fun while optimising clinical signs. Note forehead movement, which is preserved in upper motor neurone palsies but lost in lower motor neurone palsies.

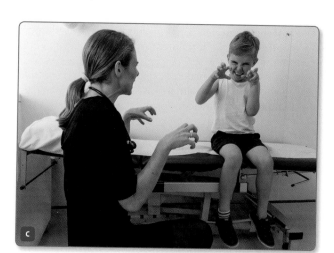

**Figure 9.5** *Continued.*

### Hearing and balance – CN VIII (vestibulocochlear)

Ask the parents whether there are problems with hearing or balance. With older children, test hearing unilaterally by rustling your fingers close to one ear while whispering in the other ear a phrase for the child to repeat. Expose younger children to soft sounds on one side while distracting them with a rattle on the other.

### Neck movements – CN XI (accessory)

Check the sternocleidomastoid muscle, which turns the head to the opposite side. Assess the trapezius muscle, which shrugs the shoulder.

### The oropharynx – CN IX, X and XII (glossopharyngeal, vagus and hypoglossal)

To test CN IX, ask older children about alterations in their sense of taste. It is hard to assess this in younger children as increased fussiness of eating has many causes (see **Chapter 13**).

CN X (vagal) nerve lesions can cause problems with swallowing. There may be a history of discoordinated swallowing or recurrent choking on feeds, suggesting a bulbar palsy. Inspect the mouth. Check the movement of the uvula: this deviates towards the side of a lesion, as tone is lost in the palate.

To examine CN XII, encourage the child to stick the tongue out – mimicry may be required. Look for deviation towards the affected side and for fasciculation of the tongue.

## Examination of the limbs

Examination of the limbs follows the scheme:

- tone
- power
- tendon reflexes
- sensation

### Tone

Tone is the degree of stiffness or flaccidity of a muscle at rest. It reflects the proportion of neuromuscular junctions that are actively transmitting acetylcholine at any one time, causing muscle to contract. In healthy muscle, tone is regulated by descending inhibition from the CNS.

If there is a brain or spinal injury, the tone to the muscles controlled by that region of the CNS increases because descending inhibition is lost. This results in a stiff or spastic muscle (hypertonia).

If there is an injury to a peripheral nerve innervating a muscle, no impulses can reach the neuromuscular junction, and the muscle fibres are not activated. This results in a floppy, weak muscle (hypotonia), sometimes with fasciculations.

The examination strategy depends on the age of the child.

**Infants**  With the child lying down, pull them up by their hands (**Figure 9.6**) so they are sitting; watch the head position. By around 3–4 months of age, healthy infants bring the head up quickly to a position in line with the trunk. A significant lag of the head behind the body after the age of 4 months suggests hypotonia.

**All children**  Gently hold the child's limbs and flex and extend the main joints. A hypertonic limb offers resistance as the joint is flexed and extended. Ask the child to relax if they can. A normal limb should be loose but not feel like a rag doll's.

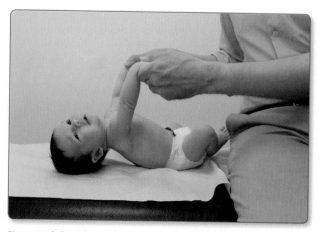

**Figure 9.6** Pulling a baby up to sit. The head lag is normal for this 10-day-old baby, but is concerning in a 4-month-old child.

Check for clonus (rhythmic, beating contractions) by holding the leg and, with the other hand, rapidly dorsiflexing the relaxed ankle. Clonus is seen and felt in the calf muscles if there is hypertonia.

### Power

For infants and non-mobile children, power is inferred during the developmental assessment by looking at head lag, trunk control, hand preference and mobility (see **Chapter 5**).

Power is measured in older children (about 5 years of age and older) using the Medical Research Council grading system (**Table 9.8**).

Power in all the muscle groups can be tested by playing 'strength games' using the following script:

### Arms

- 'Put your arms up like a chicken!'
- Place your hands on the child's elbows.
- 'Now stop me pushing your wings down.'
- 'Stop me pushing your wings up.'
- 'Put your hands up like a boxer.'

| Power | Grade |
|---|---|
| Normal power against resistance | 5 |
| Some movement against resistance, normal antigravity movement | 4 |
| No movement against resistance but can overcome gravity | 3 |
| Movement possible, but not against gravity | 2 |
| Visible contraction but no movement at a joint | 1 |
| No muscle contraction visible | 0 |

Table 9.8 Medical Research Council grading of muscle power

Stablise the elbow with one hand and hold the child's fist with your other.
- 'Push me away from you. Now the other side.'
- 'Pull me towards you. Now the other side.'
- 'Spread your fingers apart into stars.'
- 'Stop me squeezing them together.'
- 'Hold your hands out like you're holding a pizza.'
- 'Now close your eyes. Keep them closed.'

Observe for sinking of the arms on one side. This is pronator drift, a sensitive marker of intracranial pathology.
- 'Now make quacking ducks with your hands. Keep the ducks' mouths open.'

The child should be holding the four fingers of each hand parallel to each other, with the thumb at 90°.
- 'Now stop me pushing the ducks' beaks.'

The child should resist lateral pressure placed on the thumb. The 'duck's head' shape is the easiest way to get a child to position their thumb correctly for this test.

### Legs
- 'Sit on the floor. Now get up and climb on to on the couch.'
- 'Lie still. Now stop me lifting your leg in the air. Now the other side.'

Place your hand under each leg in turn and try to raise it off the bed.
- 'Lift your leg into the air against me. Now the other side.'

Press down on the thigh, each thigh in turn.
- 'Now pull your heel in towards your bottom.'

Stabilise the knee with one hand and place the other behind the heel. Pull against the child's effort.
- 'Now push me away with your foot.'
- 'Legs straight now. Pull your toes up to point at your nose.

Watch the foot and toes hyperextend and push against them with your hand.

> **Clinical insight**
>
> A child who gets up by placing the hands on the thighs to help push themselves up (Gower's sign) has proximal muscle weakness, indicative of muscular dystrophy.

### Tendon reflexes

The techniques for eliciting the deep tendon reflexes in children are the same as those used in adults. The reflexes can usually be elicited even in a young baby with the right amount of persuasion, distraction and gentle handling, and with experience and practice.

Ensure that the child is relaxed. Place your index finger over the tendon and then slowly let the tendon hammer fall on your finger. The reflex may be easier to elicit if the child clenches the teeth just as the exposed tendon is struck with the tendon hammer. Test all the deep tendons:
- patellar tendon
- gastrocnemius tendon
- bicipital tendon in the elbow
- triceps tendon behind the elbow
- brachioradialis tendon at the wrist

Watch the muscle that is supposed to contract. It should contract quickly and then relax. It may be possible to feel the contraction through your index finger more easily than visualising it, especially in obese children.

> **Clinical insight**
>
> Demonstrate the tendon reflexes on yourself and a parent first. Standing over a child with a hammer can scare them: make it funny so that the child wants a turn.

Reduced reflexes or areflexia is a worrying sign of spinal or lower motor neurone pathology (**Table 9.9**). Hyperreflexia suggests an intracranial or higher spinal pathology.

| Unilateral or localised conditions | Bilateral or generalised conditions |
|---|---|
| Spinal tumour<br>Disc protrusion (rare in children)<br>Syringomyelia<br>Acute myelitis | Spinal muscular atrophy<br>Peripheral neuropathy, e.g. Guillain–Barré syndrome |

**Table 9.9** Causes of loss of a deep tendon reflex

## Sensation

Five modalities of sensation can be tested in the limbs:

- light touch, tested with cotton wool
- sharp touch and pain, tested with a blunt neurology pin or an 'orange stick'
- vibration, tested with a tuning fork of pain and heat sensation
- joint position (proprioception) tested by moving the child's joints with the child's eyes closed
- temperature, using a cold spray or warm hands

Each sensory modality corresponds to a different type of sensory fibre with a different size and different neural pathway (**Table 9.10**).

## Cerebellar examination

The cerebellum is responsible for coordinating motor movements. Most children >4 years of age, and some slightly younger ones, can manage these tests if compliant and engaged. The mnemonic **DANISH**, which describes different cerebellar impairments, offers a way to structuring the examination.

> ## Clinical insight
>
> Hypoxia starves nerve cells of oxygen in order from largest to smallest. Therefore movement is lost before light touch, then proprioception and then vibration, temperature and pain. Local anaesthetics starve nerves of their electric potentials in the opposite order. So low doses create a loss of pain and heat sensation. Much higher doses are required to disrupt myelinated cold, firm touch or movement fibres.

**Dysdiadochokinesia** This is the inability to perform rapidly alternating movements. If the child is able, get them to repeatedly pronate and supinate one hand on the other hand, and then reverse the hands.

| Sensation | Fibre | Anatomical pathway |
|-----------|-------|--------------------|
| Light touch | Myelinated Aβ | Dorsal column medial lemniscus tract |
| Sharp touch/pain | Thinly myelinated Aδ and unmyelinated C | Lateral spinothalamic tract |
| Vibration | Myelinated Aβ and thinly myelinated Aδ | Anterior spinothalamic tract |
| Proprioception | Myelinated Aα | Dorsal column medial lemniscus tract |
| Heat | Unmyelinated C | Lateral spinothalamic tract |
| Cold | Thinly myelinated Aδ | Lateral spinothalamic tract |

**Table 9.10** Sensory fibres and their anatomical pathways

### Clinical insight

Toddlers naturally have a broad unsteady gait. Assessing the under-3s for ataxia is done better through the history. Ask about regression in feeding, grasping, drawing and walking, which require coordinated movement.

Dysdiadochokinesia can be elicited in speech by asking the child to repeat 'pat-a-cake, pat-a-cake' over and over. Younger children may be clumsier than normal when doing star-jumps, high-fiving or clapping.

**Ataxia**   Look for a broad-based gait when walking. When the child is lying down, ask them to rub their ankle up and down the opposite shin.

**Nystagmus**   Repeat the finger/toy-following test used for CN III, IV and VI (see page 168), but look for beating lateral movements of the eyes. There are sometimes visible at rest, but are more easily seen on quick lateral eye movements.

**Intention tremor**   Watch the child pick up small objects. An ataxic child has a stark tremor on reaching out. Engage the child in high-fiving, and note whether they miss your hand. A more sensitive test is the finger–nose test. Hold your index finger at the child's arm length from their face and ask them to quickly touch their nose and then your finger. Move your finger around to judge how the child performs in different areas of the visual field. Remember to test both their arms.

**Speech difficulty** Engage the child in conversation. They may have developed a new stammer or have become dysarthric

**Hypotonia** Recall your examination of the tone in all four limbs.

> ## Clinical insight
>
> It is an oversimplification to state that 'the right hand side of the brain controls the left hand side of the body' and vice versa. Unlike cortical lesions, cerebellar lesions produce ipsilateral, not contralateral, clinical signs. Therefore a left hypertonic arm with brisk reflexes suggests right-sided cortical pathology, but a left-sided hypotonic arm with an intention tremor suggests a left-sided cerebellar lesion.

### Primitive reflexes

The primitive reflexes are present at birth and should have disappeared by 4 months of age. Persistence beyond 6 months of age (corrected for prematurity) indicates serious pathology. These reflexes include the:

- Moro reflex
- asymmetrical tonic neck reflex
- rooting and sucking reflexes
- grasp reflex
- stepping reflex
- plantar reflex

These reflexes form part of the neonatal check (see **Chapter 2**).

**Moro 'startle' reflex** With the infant lying prone; gently lift up the head and then suddenly allow the head to drop a short distance (see page 31). Look for an initial symmetrical abduction of the arms, often accompanied by a startled look on the baby's face, that is followed by arm adduction. Asymmetry is concerning.

**Asymmetrical tonic neck reflex**  With the baby lying prone, gently turn the head to one side by placing the palm of one hand on the side of the head. As the head turns, the ipsilateral arm and leg extend outwards towards the direction of the head while the contralateral limbs flexes. This is known as the fencer's, archer's or 'superhero' posture. The baby usually adopts this posture for only a few seconds.

## Clinical insight

Do not test the swimming reflex. This is the paddling movement of the arms and legs when a baby is placed face down into water. It is obviously unsafe to do and is not diagnostically helpful.

**Rooting and sucking reflexes**  When you stroke the side of the infant's mouth, the infant will turn their head to try to suck your finger; this is 'rooting'.

Allow the baby to suck your finger. They will suck vigorously, at least until realising that there is no milk coming out.

**Grasp reflex**  Stroke the palm or sole with a finger. The baby will flex the fingers or toes to grasp your finger. If the baby's hand or foot is already in the flexed position, gently stroke the dorsal aspect of the hand or foot, and it will be extended.

**Stepping reflex**  Hold the baby upright, gently dangling above the bed, and then slowly bring them down until the feet touch the bed. They will make an attempt at stepping.

**Plantar reflex**  Firmly stroke upwards along the plantar fascia with a smooth object or gloved thumb. In children <4 months of age, it is normal for the big toe to curl upwards. In older children, such a response is referred to as the Babinski sign and suggests upper motor neurone pathology.

## 9.4 Examination summary

A summary of the neurological examination is given in **Table 9.11**.

| Component | Key findings |
|---|---|
| General assessment | Dysmorphia, head circumference, conscious level, neurocutaneous markers |
| Mobility | Gait, mobility aids, posture, dyskinesias |
| Cranial nerves | Strabismus, nystagmus, pupil responses, sensations, face and neck movement, tongue and throat |
| Limb tone | Hypertonia, hypotonia, fasciculations |
| Limb power | Weakness, contractures |
| Deep tendon reflexes | Hyperreflexia, hypo/areflexia |
| Sensation | Light touch, sharp touch, vibration, proprioception, temperature |
| Cerebellar function | Dysdiadochokinesis, dysarthria, past-pointing, ataxia |
| Infant reflexes | Retention of primitive reflexes, non-development of protective reflexes |
| Have you ruled out … ? | Intracranial tumour, meningoencephalitis, spinal tumour, demyelination, developmental regression |

**Table 9.11** Summary of the paediatric neurological examination

# The musculoskeletal system

## chapter 10

Musculoskeletal problems, such as infection, inflammation, cancer and wear, are more complicated to diagnose and manage in children because the musculoskeletal system is still developing, a process that can itself be painful. Anatomical features alter significantly as a child grows, and this predisposes the child to different pathologies at different ages; therefore one seemingly simple symptom, painful movement, can be caused by a wide range of disease processes.

## 10.1 Clinical scenarios

### A girl no longer moving her arm

A 17-month-old girl is brought into the emergency department because she has stopped using her left arm. She is holding the arm extended and close to her body. The parents cannot recall a traumatic injury, but there was an episode in the supermarket last night when she refused to get up from the floor. When they pulled her up firmly by the hand, she started to cry.

#### Differential diagnosis
This includes:
- a fracture of the humerus, elbow or forearm
- a pulled (subluxed) elbow

#### Further information
The arm is held extended and adducted, but the child does not seem to be distressed. Inspection of the limb shows no swelling or redness. There is no tenderness in any part of the limb. Flexion of the elbow is resisted.

#### Conclusion
With no clear trauma other than the pulling injury, and no clinical abnormalities of swelling or tenderness, a subluxed elbow is most likely. This can easily be relocated.

## Acute limp

A 30-month-old boy woke up with a left-sided limp and is reluctant to bear weight on that side. He is complaining of pain but cannot point to the precise source. There is no history of trauma. He has recently had a mild cold. There is no history of fevers, and vital signs, including temperature are normal. He is happy apart from the pain when walking.

### Differential diagnosis

This includes:

- irritable hip (transient synovitis)
- septic arthritis
- fracture
- leukaemia

### Further information

The boy looks well, happy and alert. He is lying on the couch with his left leg semi-flexed and externally rotated. There is no fever or rash. The leg is not red or swollen, and palpation reveals no tenderness or increased warmth. There is no pallor or unexplained bruising. The child has been eating and drinking well.

Passive examination of the hip reveals slightly reduced flexion, normal external rotation, abduction and adduction, but significantly reduced internal rotation, which causes a lot of pain.

### Conclusion

The most likely diagnosis is an irritable hip that will spontaneously resolve. Although septic arthritis is possible, the normal vital signs and temperature are inconsistent with this. The lack of trauma and bony tenderness makes a fracture unlikely. The normal colour and appetite, as well as the localisation of pain to joint movement rather than bone, helps to rule out leukaemia.

## A girl who is not weightbearing

An 18-month-old girl has had a swollen right ankle for the past 4 days. The ankle has become increasingly warm and tender, and she refuses to bear weight on the affected side. There was a minor injury 10 days ago when she tripped over a toy on the floor. However, there are now fevers of up to 39°C, and the child is not wanting to eat.

## Differential diagnosis

This includes:

- septic arthritis
- reactive arthritis
- osteomyelitis
- fracture

## Further information

The toddler appears unwell, irritable and miserable. The right ankle is swollen and tender to palpation. It is warm and there is overlying erythema. There is reduced movement of the ankle.

## Conclusion

The most urgent differential diagnosis to exclude is septic arthritis because it rapidly causes permanent joint damage, and deterioration into systemic sepsis can be both rapid and fatal. Blood samples for culture should be taken immediately and antibiotics started before any results come back. They can always be stopped if test results are negative. Ultrasound will identify a joint effusion, and this should be followed by formal exploration under general anaesthetic.

# 10.2 Common presentations

Key musculoskeletal presentations in children include:

- acute limp
- single joint swelling
- polyarthritis

## Acute limp

A new limp should be treated as a potential malignancy or infection until proven otherwise. As well as neurological problems (see **Chapter 9**), there are many musculoskeletal causes (**Table 10.1**).

| Pathology | Example(s) |
|---|---|
| Trauma | Fractures, soft tissue injuries |
| Infection | Septic arthritis, osteomyelitis |
| Inflammation | Transient synovitis |
| Bone destruction | Perthes' disease, slipped upper femoral epiphysis, rickets |
| Autoimmune | Juvenile arthritis, systemic lupus erythematosus |
| Infiltrations | Haemarthrosis, haemochromatosis |
| Malignancy | Leukaemia, osteosarcoma |

**Table 10.1** Causes of acute limp

Limp is commonly caused by trauma, including 'toddler fracture' and buckle fracture:

- A toddler fracture is a spiral fracture, usually of the distal tibia, caused by a simple twisting injury. It is often unnoticed if the mechanism of injury seems mild.
- Buckle fractures are caused by falling onto an outstretched limb and are often missed on radiographs because there is no obvious crack through the periosteum (**Figure 10.1**).

## Clinical insight

A child should not be considered to be 'limping' until you have seen them limp in bare feet. Ill-fitting footwear or a foreign body in the shoe should be excluded to save unnecessary investigation.

### Transient synovitis

Transient synovitis (also known as irritable hip) is a common condition in toddlers and younger children (3–10 years of age). It is usually a reactive synovitis in response to a recent viral infection, often a simple cold. If there is a joint effusion, it is sterile, with no organisms seen on microscopy.

It can present in a similar way to septic arthritis so the two are easily confused.

*Clinical features*  Unlike children with septic arthritis, those with transient synovitis are systemically well and often afebrile. There is a history of preceding viral infection. The child

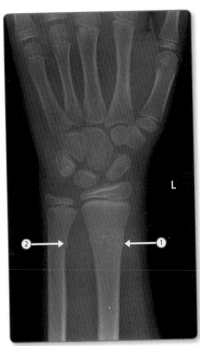

**Figure 10.1** A buckle fracture of the radius and greenstick fracture of the ulna. Note ① the distortion of the radial periostium without an obvious crack and ② the small crack within the periosteum of the ulna.

may hold the hip in a flexed position at rest and resist passive movement of the affected hip.

## Septic arthritis

Septic arthritis is caused by a bacterial infection of the joint capsule. Bacteria reach the joint via direct spread from adjacent osteomyelitis or by haematogenous spread. Other causes are trauma and clinical procedures, for example joint aspiration.

*Clinical features*  Signs and symptoms of septic arthritis are:

- fever and tachycardia
- joint swelling, warmth and erythema (these may be difficult to assess in the hip)
- joint pain (arthralgia) on active and passive movement

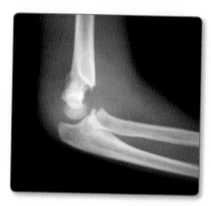

**Figure 10.2** Chronic osteomyelitis in the elbow, which has affected bone growth.

- restriction of joint movement as a result of the pain

Infections of the musculoskeletal system are more frequent in younger children (<8 years) and are usually caused by *Staphylococcus aureus* or *Streptococcus pyogenes*. Delay in treatment can cause permanent joint or bone damage, affecting growth (**Figure 10.2**).

## Osteomyelitis

Osteomyelitis is an infection of bone, usually the metaphysis of long bones. It is more common in children with sickle cell disease, in whom a minority of cases are caused by *Salmonella* or *Kingella* spp. rather than the more typical *Staphylococcus* or *Streptococcus* spp.

*Clinical features*  Infants and toddlers with osteomyelitis present with:
- non-specific symptoms of feeling or seeming unwell
- poor feeding
- fever, which is often low grade
- restriction of movement in the affected limb
- crying and discomfort when the limb is moved or palpated

## Perthes' disease

Perthes' disease is an idiopathic avascular necrosis of the femoral head. This causes deformity and flattening of the head of the

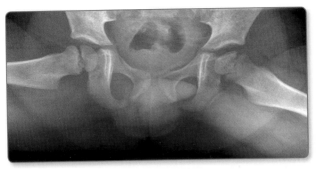

**Figure 10.3** Perthes' disease (avascular necrosis of the femoral head). Note the normal growth plate at the head of the right femur, and the abnormal appearance at the head of the left femur.

femur (**Figure 10.3**), which can lead to osteoarthritis in later life. It occurs in younger children (3–8 years of age) and affects boys more than girls.

> ## Clinical insight
>
> Limb pain is a common feature of meningococcal sepsis. Microvascular ischaemia causes agonising pain, which can present hours before the characteristic non-blanching rash.

*Clinical features* Perthes' disease presents with:

- an indolent course, over a few weeks
- aching pain at rest
- restriction of active and passive movement of the affected hip
- preservation of leg length
- antalgic gait
- referred pain to the knee

## Slipped upper femoral epiphysis

In this condition, the proximal femur slips at the growth plate, so the epiphysis stays in the acetabular socket while the metaphysis moves superiorly and anteriorly (**Figure 10.4**). It classically affects overweight teenagers and is more common in boys.

*Clinical features* Symptoms and signs of are similar to those of a fractured neck of femur:

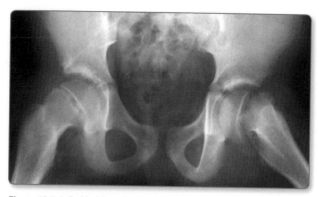

**Figure 10.4** Left-sided slipped upper femoral epiphysis.

- pain in the hip or knee
- antalgic or waddling gait
- discrepancy in leg length, the affected leg being shorter
- a hip joint that is held in external rotation

## Malignancy

Malignancy affects children of all ages and, although rare, must always be considered. Cancers of the musculoskeletal system present as a tumour of the bone (osteosarcoma), muscle (rhabdomyosarcoma) or marrow (leukaemia). Marrow proliferation raises pressure inside the bone and therefore causes pain similar to that of osteomyelitis.

*Clinical features*　As well as bone pain, signs of potential malignancy include:

- pallor from anaemia
- easy bruising from thrombocytopenia
- fracture from low-impact trauma
- weight loss and loss of appetite

## Single joint swelling

As well as being caused by trauma and infection, swelling in a single joint can be caused by:

- reactive arthritis
- haemarthrosis

## Reactive arthritis

Reactive arthritis can occur after viral and bacterial infections. The effusion itself is sterile despite there being an infection elsewhere. Reactive arthritis is thought to occur when antibodies against a current infection also bind to synovial tissue.

*Clinical features*  The presenting features of reactive and septic arthritis are similar, so they are often confused. The main features of reactive arthritis are:

- a history of preceding infection (often gastrointestinal)
- joint swelling and effusion
- arthralgia
- restriction of movement

## Haemarthrosis

The two main causes are haemophilia and trauma, often including a ligamentous tear (e.g. of the anterior cruciate ligament).

*Clinical features*  Haemarthrosis often features:

- a history of trauma
- significant joint swelling
- bruising around the joint
- pain with restricted joint movement

## Polyarthritis

Polyarthritis is relatively uncommon in childhood. There are a wide variety of rare causes, but two which cause severe problems the longer they go undiagnosed are:

- juvenile idiopathic arthritis
- rheumatic fever

## Juvenile idiopathic arthritis

This is the most common cause of polyarthritis (inflammation of five or more joints) in childhood. It is less common as a cause of oligoarthritis (four or fewer joints affected). There are many different subtypes, which are beyond the scope of this book.

It is more common in children with pre-existing autoimmune conditions, including type 1 diabetes.

*Clinical features*  The presentation depends on the subset, but generally it involves:

- a chronic course of ≥6 weeks
- joint pain and swelling, with some restriction of function
- pain and stiffness that is worse in the morning and eases as the day progresses
- fevers, a pale pink rash, hepatosplenomegaly and lethargy in systemic-onset disease
- psoriasis in psoriatic juvenile idiopathic arthritis
- a family history of autoimmune disease

## Clinical insight

When polyarthritis presents with other symptoms, always test for antinuclear antibody, complement fractions, antiphospholipid antibody and haemolysis. These may suggest a diagnosis of systemic lupus erythematosus rather than juvenile idiopathic arthritis (**Table 10.2**).

### Rheumatic fever

Rheumatic fever is uncommon in developed countries but it is still seen in developing ones. It is an immune complication of *Streptococcus* infection, often tonsillitis. The immune reaction affects many tissues, including the heart, causing carditis; this leads to fibrosis and valve disease, particularly mitral stenosis.

*Clinical features*  Rheumatic fever is diagnosed using the Duckett Jones criteria (**Table 10.3**). The diagnosis is made if there is evidence of recent *Streptococcus* infection (raised anti-streptolysin O titre or positive culture) together with either two major criteria, or one major and two minor criteria.

### Growing pains

Growing pains are very common and can be severe. They are, however, a diagnosis of exclusion. They usually occur in children undergoing 'growth spurts'.

*Clinical features*  Growing pains are usually bilateral, aching, intermittent pains in long bones. They wax and wane. In teenagers, severe pain can be caused by fragmentation of the

| Symptomatic criteria | Laboratory criteria |
|---|---|
| Cutaneous lupus | Positive antinuclear antibody |
| Oral/nasal ulceration | Positive anti-dsDNA antibody |
| Alopecia | Positive anti-smooth muscle |
| Arthritis | antibody |
| Serositis | Low complement |
| Nephritis | Positive antiphospholipid antibody |
| Neurological abnormality | Positive Coombs' test |
| Haemolysis | |
| Low white blood cell count | |
| Thrombocytopenia | |
| dsDNA, double-stranded DNA | |

**Table 10.2** American College of Rheumatology diagnostic criteria for systemic lupus erythematosus. At least four criteria, including one from each column, are required for a diagnosis of systemic lupus erythematosus

| Major criteria | Minor criteria |
|---|---|
| Carditis | Fever |
| Polyarthritis (migrating) | Arthralgia |
| Erythema marginatum | PR interval prolongation on ECG |
| Subcutaneous nodules | Raised erythrocyte sedimentation |
| Sydenham's chorea | rate or C-reactive protein |
| | Raised leucocyte count |
| | Previous history of rheumatic fever |

**Table 10.3** Duckett Jones criteria for diagnosis of rheumatic fever

tibial tubercle during growth spurts, particularly in boys. This is Osgood–Schlatter's disease (**Figure 10.5**), which, although usually benign and self-limiting, can predispose to avulsion fractures (**Figure 10.5a**).

# 10.3 Examination of the musculoskeletal system

Just as you would not examine only one lobe of the lung, you should not restrict your examination to only one joint. A thorough musculoskeletal examination must include the affected

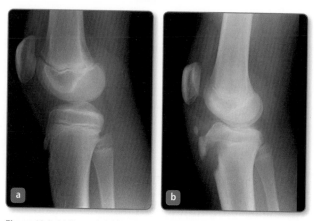

**Figure 10.5** (a) Osgood–Schlatter's disease. (b) Avulsion fracture of the tibial tubercle in Osgood–Schlatter's disease.

joint, the joint above, the joint below and the joint opposite, as pain can be referred from one site to the other.

A sequence for examining musculoskeletal function is:

- general inspection
- 'look, feel, move'
- paediatric 'gait, arms, legs and spine' (pGALS) examination
- focused assessment of specific joints
- assessment of trauma
- assessment for child maltreatment

## General inspection

Stand back and observe the child. Watching a playing child from a distance provides valuable clues. Jumping in too early may also frighten the child and lose you the opportunity to elicit pertinent signs.

Before the focused assessment, observe:

- gait and limb use – which shows the impact of the problem
- growth and nutritional state –as chronic musculoskeletal problems affect growth
- joint deformity – which may be obvious from a distance
- rashes – e.g. psoriasis, malar rashes, eczema and cellulitis

- orthotic aids – e.g. splints and crutches
- ethnicity – as children with darker skin have a greater risk of developing rickets
- lethargy and pallor – which may suggest malignancy

## 'Look, feel, move'

The 'look, feel, move' approach is the gold standard for detecting clinical signs in joints.

### Look

Observe the following:

- posture
- guarding
- deformity
- swelling
- erythema
- bruising
- active movement

**Posture**  You may see clues in the child's posture:

- A child who has an acute scoliosis may have an inflammatory intra-abdominal lesion.
- A child who is holding the arm extended, parallel to the body and internally rotated is exhibiting the classic sign of a 'pulled' elbow

**Guarding**  If the child is holding their hand over an affected area, this suggests a significant injury to the protected area.

**Deformity**  This can give a clue to an underlying pathology, including fracture. Muscle wasting suggests prolonged underuse, possibly due to pain.

A comparison of leg lengths can provide clues, for example to distinguish Perthes' disease from slipped upper femoral epiphysis. Use a tape measure to confirm the lengths.

**Swelling**  Joint swelling suggests an effusion, but a mid-limb swelling may indicate a fracture or bone tumour. Swelling can be subtle. Compare the affected limb with the contralateral limb. The hip joint, lying deep, is not easily assessed for swelling.

**Erythema**  This is a non-specific sign, but may represent:
- cellulitis
- early bruising
- septic arthritis
- osteomyelitis
- inflammatory arthritis

**Bruising**  This signposts a possible underlying injury. A bruise goes through a number of colour changes, the timing of which is highly variable. There is no evidence that the colour of a bruise can be used to 'age' it accurately, and attempts to do so have led to difficulties during child protection investigations.

Look for bruises on multiple areas of the body. Their locations may give evidence of easy bruising (over bony prominences) or of child maltreatment (non-bony areas such as buttocks and ears).

**Active movement**  Ask the child to move the affected area to assess the full range of movements. The limited range of painful movements can be very specific, as in shoulder impingement syndrome (pain on abduction but not flexion). School-age children can follow the pGALS script); younger children can be encouraged to play and reach for toys.

Feel

Palpate the joint and assess for:
- tenderness
- temperature
- crepitus

When palpating, do not look at the joint. Instead, observe the child's face for grimacing or signs of pain. Assessment can be complicated by a child's fear of pain, rather than pain itself.

Palpate in an orderly sequence, examining the whole joint margin, and noting areas of localised tenderness. Some deep joints, such as the hip, are not amenable to full palpation. Also palpate adjacent bone and surrounding muscle.

**Temperature**  Feel the joint with the back of a hand, and compare the temperature with that of the other side. An increased temperature suggests an infection or an inflammatory joint disorder.

**Crepitus** Gently flex and extend a joint. Crepitus is felt as a 'creaking' or 'bubbling'. Its presence suggests an inflammatory or degenerative change within the joint.

**Fluid thrill** Examining for an effusion by fluid thrill is unique to the knees.

Perform a 'patellar tap' test to assess for fluid in the knee:

- Place a hand over the leg above the patella and slide it down to just above the upper border of the patella, squeezing out fluid in the suprapatellar pouch.
- With the index finger of the other hand, press over the patella.
- Palpate and observe for a 'bouncing' movement of the patella off the femur. Its presence suggests increased fluid in the joint space.

## Move

Active (patient-led) movement has already been assessed to elicit pain and guarding. Passive (clinician-led) movement detects joint restriction.

## pGALS examination

The pGALS is a modified paediatric version of the adult GALS approach to examining the musculoskeletal system; it is a screening tool which aims to elicit signs by testing all the muscles and joints of the body. Although it is suitable for use only in children who can obey commands, it can be easily turned into a series of games to help younger children comply. Videos of pGALS being used are available on the Internet.

The outline of pGALS is shown below in the form of a script.

## Gait

Look for antalgia, swinging, asymmetry and weakness:

- 'Walk to the wall and back.'
- 'Walk on your heels.'
- 'Walk on your tiptoes.'

## Arms

Look for weakness, pain, restriction and asymmetry:

- 'Put your hands out in front of you.'

- 'Turn your hand over and make a fist.'
- 'Make an 'O' with your thumb and index finger.'
- 'Now touch your thumbs with the tips of your other fingers.'
- 'Hold this piece of paper between your finger and thumb. Now don't let me pull it away.'
- 'Put your hands and wrists together' (**Figure 10.6a**).
- 'Put your hands back to back' (**Figure 10.6b**).
- 'Spread your fingers. Reach up as far as you can.'
- 'Look at the ceiling.'
- 'Put your hands behind your neck.'
- 'Now let me twiddle your fingers.' (Squeeze and rotate the child's metacarpophalangeal joints.)

## Legs

Look for weakness, pain, restriction and asymmetry. Feel for crepitus.

- 'I'm going to tap your knee.' (Perform a patellar tap).
- 'Bring your ankle up to your bottom.'
- 'Make your legs nice and floppy.' (Assess passive movement of hip and knee, including rotation).

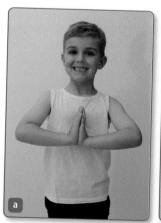
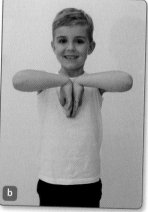

**Figure 10.6** (a) Prayer sign and (b) reverse prayer sign.

## Spine

For the pGALS examination of the spine, give the following instructions:

- 'Turn your head to the right.' 'Turn your head to the left.' 'Place your ear on your shoulder.' 'Now the other side.'
- 'Open your mouth wide and place three fingers inside.' (This assesses the temporomandibular joint.)
- 'Let me look at your back. Can you twist your body around to the left?'
- 'And now to the right.'
- 'Now bend forwards.' (Place your fingers above and below the posterior superior iliac spine. As the child bends forwards, your fingers should move apart. Then palpate for scoliosis, see **Figure 10.7**).

## Beighton score

Complete the pGALS examination with the Beighton score, which tests for hypermobility of the joints:

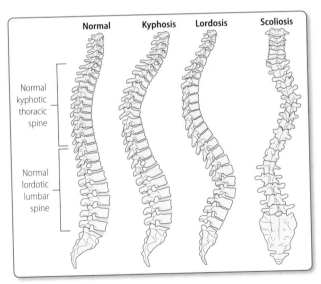

**Figure 10.7** Normal spine and spinal anomalies.

## Clinical insight

Tailor your script to the age of the child you are examining. A 4-year-old may not respond well to 'Spread your fingers'; 'reach up'; 'look at the ceiling' – but may respond better to 'make a star'; 'put it in the sky'; 'look up at it twinkling'.

- 'Can you put your hands flat on the floor with your knees straight?' (1 point)
- 'How far back can you pull your little fingers?' (1 point per side beyond 90°)
- 'Can you bend your thumb back to touch your wrist?' (1 point per side)
- 'I am going to pull your elbow backwards slightly.' (1 point per side beyond 180°)
- 'I am going to bend your knee backwards slightly.' (1 point per side beyond 180°)

A total score of 0–4 is normal. A score of 6–9 shows serious widespread ligamentous laxity. A child with a score >4 should be referred for physiotherapy and investigation to distinguish benign 'hypermobility' from a widespread connective tissue disorder such as Ehlers–Danlos syndrome.

## Focused assessment of specific joints

When a child presents with pathology in one joint, assess this joint in detail as well as screening the whole musculoskeletal system. This section relates to the spine, hips and knees.

### Spine

Assess the entire spine from cervical spine to coccyx in a logical order.

Fully expose the spine and look for deformity. Note the child's posture, 'steps' in the spine and overlying swelling or redness. Palpate for tenderness to rule out:
- an underlying fracture (if there is history of trauma)
- a muscular strain
- an alignment abnormality (e.g. spondylolisthesis)
- an infection (e.g. spinal tuberculosis or discitis)

**Cervical spine**  Check the neck posture – a cervical spine lesion may produce a head tilt, such as torticollis. A head tilt may also be compensation for an acute squint (compression of the trochlear nerve by raised intracranial pressure), so consider intracranial malignancy.

Look at the size of the neck and assess whether it appears short. A short neck can occur in certain syndromes (e.g. Turner's syndrome) and in conditions such as Klippel–Feil disease, in which there is fusion of two or more cervical vertebrae.

Assess movement. In younger children, this can be done by letting the child follow toys or bubbles by moving their head. Remember that a child may resist passive movement of the neck because of fear rather than pain.

**Thoracic spine**  Look for evidence of a scoliosis, kyphosis (**Figure 10.7**) or both. Observe flexion, extension and lateral movement of the spine, looking for restriction of movement. Most scoliosis is idiopathic (80%) or congenital, but in a minority of cases it also indicates:

- a neurological disorder, e.g. cerebral palsy or muscular dystrophy
- intra-abdominal inflammation, e.g. an appendix abscess
- a spinal tumour

**Lumbosacral spine**  Review the normal lordosis. It may be exaggerated in conditions such as muscular dystrophy, and reduced in inflammatory diseases of the lumbar spine. Observe forward flexion and extension.

Examine for pain in the sacroiliac joints by taking hold of the outer aspects of the pelvis and gently pressing inwards.

## Hip

**Approach**  Examine the gait: some disorders of the hip present with antalgia or deformity.

The hip joint is deep, so you cannot palpate it fully. Assess the six key movements of the hip, both actively and passively:

- flexion (**Figure 10.8a**) and extension
- adduction and abduction (**Figure 10.8b**)
- internal and external (**Figure 10.9**) rotation

*Appearance*  A child with an antalgic gait leans to the side of the painful hip. They take a rapid, heavy step on the painful side, followed by a slower step on the unaffected side.

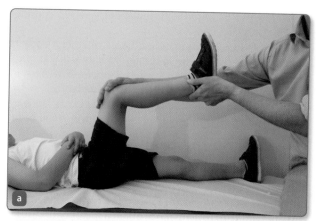

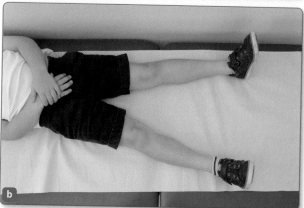

**Figure 10.8** Hip movements: (a) flexion, (b) abduction.

In the non-ambulant child, look for cessation of crawling, reduced movements on one side, and noticeable flexion and external rotation of the hip when supine. If lifted to a standing position, a child with hip effusion may keep the hip flexed, with reluctance to bear weight on the affected side.

**Associated conditions** The child's age should be noted when assessing the likely cause of hip pathology (**Table 10.4**).

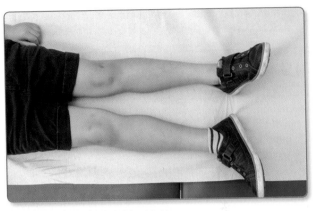

**Figure 10.9** External rotation of the right hip.

| 0–3 years of age | 3–10 years of age | >10 years of age |
|---|---|---|
| Developmental dysplasia<br>Septic arthritis<br>Osteomyelitis | Perthes' disease (avascular necrosis of the femoral head; see Figure 10.3)<br>Transient synovitis (irritable hip) | Slipped upper femoral epiphysis (see Figure 10.4)<br>Reactive arthritis<br>Avulsion fractures, e.g. anterior superior iliac spine fracture |

**Table 10.4** Guide to the most common causes of hip pain in children at different ages

The age ranges are only a guide as overlap occurs (e.g. infection of bone and joints occurs at all ages, but is most common in infants and young children).

### Knee

*Approach* Fully expose the joint and look at its position and characteristics:
- Feel the knee for tenderness – ensure you assess the medial and lateral collateral ligaments, the joint line, the tibial tuberosity and the patella.

- If there is an effusion, try to elicit a patellar tap (see **p. xxx**).
- As well as assessing flexion and extension movements, apply varus and valgus stresses with the knee straight to test for collateral ligament instability (**Figure 10.10**). Use the 'draw' and 'sag' tests to assess the cruciate ligaments for instability (**Figure 10.11**).

***Appearance***  The knee may be held in partial flexion to reduce pain at rest. If so, estimate the degree of flexion.

Internal rotation of the knee occurs in femoral anteversion, a common, self-limiting condition that is seen in young children.

Note whether there is evidence of erythema or swelling in the joint. Look at the quadriceps muscle for signs of atrophy.

***Associated conditions***  The knee may be held in flexion with acute trauma to the knee or chronic arthritis. Other positional variants are genu valgum ('knock-knees', which can cause persisting knee pain) and genu varum. Both positions are normal variants in children between 2.5 and 4.5 years old.

Restriction of knee movement may be due to acute pathology (e.g. trauma, septic arthritis or osteomyelitis) or chronic

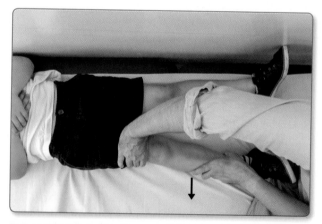

**Figure 10.10** Testing collateral ligament stability. Lateral movement of the lower leg (in the direction of the arrow) causes medial stress.

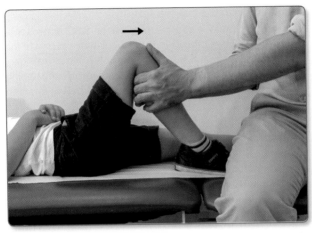

**Figure 10.11** Testing the cruciate ligaments: the anterior draw test. The patient's foot should be wedged firmly under your leg as you pull their lower leg (in the direction of the arrow). Push the knee away from you to perform the sag test.

pathology (e.g. juvenile idiopathic arthritis). In both cases, movement is restricted either by pain or (less commonly) by damage to the knee structures (e.g. a ligamentous tear or fracture).

## Clinical insight

Presentation of either muscle or bone pathology can be similar to problems with joints (e.g. psoas abscess and leukaemia, respectively). Do not restrict your examination to the joints.

### Trauma

Most children who require a musculoskeletal assessment have a history of trauma or signs suggestive of an injury. A common example is a toddler who has stopped moving their arm after being swung by their parent – a classic history for a pulled elbow, which can easily be relocated into position. To do this, to press your thumb over the radial head, while flexing the pronated arm as fully as possible. Supinate the forearm and re-extend it; a 'clunk' should be heard or felt and shortly afterwards the child will be able to move the arm normally.

### Examination in the trauma setting

In a setting of major trauma, prioritise an 'ABC' approach – assessing the Airway, Breathing and Circulation – as part of the primary survey before assessing specific joints in the secondary survey. Fractures can cause pneumothoraces or life-threatening internal bleeding, which must be controlled before focusing on pGALS.

Features indicative of a serious fracture include:
- clinical deformities (**Figure 10.12**)
- overlying skin breaches

The presence of deformity not only means that some form of manipulative treatment is needed, but also raises the possibility of neurovascular compromise. Check the pulses distal to the deformity and assess sensation: abnormal findings require urgent intervention.

An open fracture is a fracture with an overlying skin breach. A child with an open fracture should be given immediate

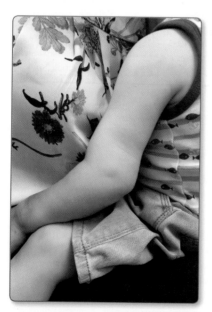

**Figure 10.12** Deformity of the left arm, with bruising.

intravenous antibiotics, and early surgery is required. There is a significant risk of osteomyelitis.

## Assessment of a fracture

The presence of growth plates in children's bones makes the diagnosis and assessment of fractures much more complicated than it is in adults. The fracture may, for example, occur through the non-ossified area – a Salter–Harris type I fracture (**Figure 10.13**). Therefore, the key to diagnosis lies in the clinical findings. A fracture is likely if there is localised tenderness over a growth plate on clinical examination, and the injury should be managed as such, even if the radiograph is normal.

**Supracondylar fracture**  This fracture above the elbow joint is one of the most common fractures associated with a risk of neurovascular compromise in children (**Figure 10.14**).

If the fracture has caused dorsal displacement of the distal bone fragment (grade III on the Gartland classification; **Figure 10.15**), the anterior proximal fragment can impinge on the brachial artery. It is crucial to palpate the radial pulse and check perfusion of the hand. If the arterial supply has been compromised, it is vital to manipulate the elbow back into position – this is usually done in the emergency department, under ketamine sedation.

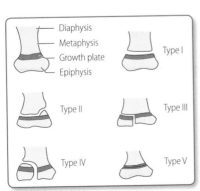

**Figure 10.13** Salter–Harris classification of fractures. Type V is a compression of the growth plate.

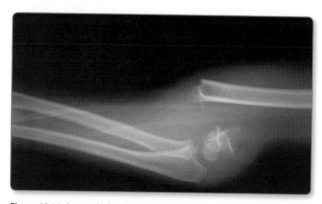

**Figure 10.14** A severely displaced supracondylar fracture. This fracture raises immediate concerns about the risk of neurovascular impairment.

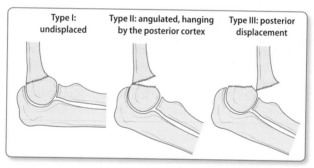

**Figure 10.15** The Gartland classification of supracondylar fractures.

Fractures of the elbow are easily misdiagnosed. The elbow joint gradually coalesces with age from multiple ossification centres so a separate bony mass on a radiograph may be a normal ossification centre rather than a bone fragment (**Figure 10.16**). **Table 10.5** details the ages at which the ossification centres fuse.

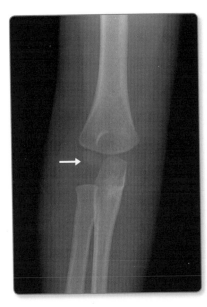

**Figure 10.16** A normal radiograph in a 2-year-old child. The arrow points not to a dislocated radial head growth plate, but to a normal ossification centre.

| Ossification centre | Age (years) |
|---|---|
| Capitellum | 1 |
| Radial head | 3 |
| Internal (medial) epicondyle | 5 |
| Trochlear | 7 |
| Olecranon | 9 |
| Lateral epicondyle | 11 |
| Use the mnemonic CRITOL to remember the ossification centres of the elbow. | |

**Table 10.5** Age at which ossification centres in the elbow should no longer be visible as separate entities on radiographs

## Child maltreatment

Children who have been maltreated often present with symptoms or signs involving the skeleton in the absence of a declared history of trauma. A high index of suspicion should be maintained. However, it should also be kept in mind that accidental injury does occur in the absence of a clear history, for example in osteogenesis imperfecta ('brittle bone disease') or a 'toddler fracture' (see page 183).

## Do not assume

You must assess unexplained injuries carefully and non-judgementally. No injury can indicate without doubt that a child has been abused, but some injuries are more likely to have been inflicted than gained accidentally, for example a long bone fracture in a non-ambulant child or multiple rib fractures.

If a significant injury is present but no mechanism of trauma is offered, the possibility of child maltreatment must be fully investigated. You must immediately inform senior staff, document the concerns. Discussions with the parents or carers about concerns regarding possible child abuse should be conducted by the most senior doctor present, and be balanced by the possibility that telling the parents may increase the risk to the child (as they may abscond with the child).

## Look further

If a fracture might have been inflicted, undertake a careful assessment of the whole skeleton by clinical examination and radiography (a skeletal survey). These can detect old and current fractures: the presence of multiple fractures of varying ages is highly suspicious of physical abuse.

Examine the child carefully for bruises. Distinguish bruises in expected places (e.g. shins) from those in unusual places (e.g. the backs of the legs or earlobes). In babies and toddlers, use fundoscopy to look for retinal haemorrhages, which can be a sign of shaking injuries.

## 10.4 Examination summary

A summary of the musculoskeletal examination is given in
**Table 10.6**.

| Component | Key findings |
|---|---|
| General Inspection | Pallor, bruising, rashes, movement, general health, posture, gait, deformities |
| pGALS | Widespread/focussed pathology, hypermobility |
| Focused inspection of joint | Scars, swelling, discoloration, deformity, wasting, guarding |
| Joint palpation | Tenderness, size, temperature, stability, effusions, crepitus |
| Movement | Passive, active, range |
| Measurement | Height plot, weight plot, leg length disparity |
| Comparison | Pathology in joints above, below and opposite |
| Neurovascular | In trauma: absent pulses, absent sensation |
| Have you ruled out … ? | Infection, malignancy, child maltreatment |
| pGALS, paediatric 'gait, arms, legs and spine'. | |

**Table 10.6** Summary of the musculoskeletal examination

# The head and neck

Examination of the ears, nose and throat is one of the hardest examinations to perform in a non-compliant child. Use of an otoscope and tongue depressor is uncomfortable and frighteningly invasive for many children. When this is added to palpation of the neck by placing the hands near the child's throat, it is easy to see why many healthcare practitioners struggle to elicit head and neck signs in children. Despite this, examination of the head and neck is among the most important skills required in paediatric clinical examination.

Many conditions present with swelling in the face, head or neck. Renal pathologies lie alongside haematological diagnoses in this chapter, but this emphasises how sensitive the head and neck area is in identifying both local and systemic disease.

Tonsillitis and ear infections remain the most common presentations in children <5 years of age. These can have severe complications: abscesses, scarlet fever and mastoiditis are still regularly seen in developed countries. Parents are often most concerned by masses and swellings. Many are benign but the distinction between malignant masses, abscesses and endocrine causes can be difficult.

## 11.1 Clinical scenarios

### Sore throat and a rash

A 4-year-old girl is brought to her GP by her mother. The girl has been having fevers and not eating much for the past 2 days.

#### Differential diagnosis

This includes:

- otitis media
- tonsillitis
- pneumonia
- urinary tract infection
- gastroenteritis

### Further information

The girl looks well and is sitting on her mother's knee. There is no significant previous medical history and the child is fully immunised. She has had a cough. There is no history of urinary symptoms, vomiting or diarrhoea.

The girl's skin is not red, but on her trunk and back it feels rough, like sandpaper. Her breath is malodorous. There is no tachypnoea, and the chest is clear on auscultation. Ear examination is normal, but throat examination shows bilaterally enlarged tonsils with exudates. A urine dipstick is negative.

### Conclusion

The girl has scarlet fever, a notifiable disease in the UK, caused by group A streptococcal tonsillitis. The appropriate public health body is notified, and a 10-day course of oral phenoxymethylpenicillin is prescribed.

## Sore ear

A 10-year-old boy comes to the emergency department with his schoolteacher. He has been complaining of ear pain for a day, and he vomited at school today after feeling dizzy.

### Differential diagnosis
This includes:
- acute otitis media
- otitis externa
- mastoiditis

### Further information

There is pus in the right ear canal, which prevents the tympanic membrane from being seen. On inspection of the face, the right ear looks to be sticking out further than the left. The skin behind the right ear is red and exquisitely tender.

### Conclusion

The boy has mastoiditis. CT will confirm the diagnosis. He should be admitted for a course of intravenous antibiotics and review by an ear, nose and throat (ENT) surgeon.

# 11.2 Common presentations

Common presentations in the head and neck include:

- facial or eye swelling
- painful ear
- sore throat
- epistaxis
- neck lumps

## Facial or eye swelling

Diffuse or focal oedema on the face is concerning and has a wide differential diagnosis:

- allergy
- nephrotic syndrome
- mumps
- conjunctivitis
- periorbital and orbital cellulitis

## Allergy

Facial swelling in acute allergy results from systemic histamine release by mast cells. The eyelids and lips are particularly sensitive areas (**Figure 11.1**).

*Clinical features*   Exposure to an allergen often produces tingling of the tongue and lips, and nausea. Swelling is either very swift or indolent. There is often a widespread itchy urticarial rash (see page 242 and Figure 12.4) and there may be difficulty breathing, with wheeze or stridor.

## Nephrotic syndrome

This is a syndrome of facial oedema and ascites caused by micro-albumin loss secondary to renal inflammation. The podocytes of the glomerulus separate, allowing protein to filter out of the blood. This results in hypoalbuminaemia and subcutaneous extravascular fluid retention ('third-spacing'). It often relapses.

*Clinical features*   Dipstick tests show proteinuria of 3+ or more, which may have produced foaming turbid urine. There is oedema, most noticeable on the face (**Figure 11.2**), that

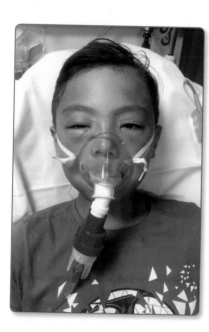

**Figure 11.1** Mucosal swelling caused by allergy to horse dander.

gradually progresses to include the abdomen (Figure 8.5), genitals and eventually the whole body. Despite looking oedematous, the child may be intravascularly hypovolaemic, with hypotension and tachycardia. This intravascular dehydration can lead to thrombosis and stroke.

## Mumps

Mumps is a viral infection that causes painful swelling of the parotid gland. It is caused by a paramyxovirus, against which there is an effective vaccine. Before vaccination, mumps was responsible for around 10% of cases of viral meningitis.

*Clinical features* There is a viral prodrome of flu-like illness, with headache, fever and malaise. Painful parotid swelling then develops. This is unilateral or bilateral and lasts 7–10 days. There are many potential side effects of mumps infection:

- meningitis
- encephalitis

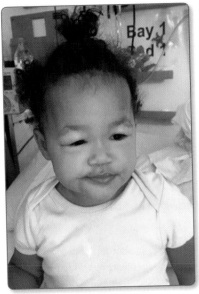

**Figure 11.2** Facial oedema in nephrotic syndrome.

- sensorineural deafness
- orchitis
- infertility
- ovarian inflammation
- pancreatitis

## Conjunctivitis

Inflammation of the conjunctivae is usually caused by viral infections (commonly adenovirus). However, bacterial conjunctivitis is also quite common (e.g. *Neisseria gonorrhoeae* or *Chlamydia trachomatis* in neonates, and staphylococci in older children). Conjunctivitis may also be an allergic phenomenon, commonly as part of the symptoms of hay fever.

***Clinical features***  Conjunctivitis presents with erythema of the conjunctivae, which is best seen over the sclera. There is often an exudate, which may be purulent.

**Clinical insight**

Neonates may have sticky yellow eyes that have an appearance similar to that of conjunctivitis. However, this is more often caused by incomplete canalisation of the nasolacrimal duct. Simple saline washes are required.

There should not be a reduction in visual acuity as a result of conjunctivitis. If this occurs, seek another cause, for example anterior uveitis, which is seen in connective tissue disorders.

### Periorbital cellulitis

Periorbital (also known as 'preseptal') cellulitis is inflammation of the tissues surrounding the eye, including the eyelids. It is caused by bacterial infection, most commonly by *Staphylococcus aureus*.

***Clinical features*** Children with preseptal cellulitis present with:
- swelling
- erythema
- tenderness of the tissues surrounding the eye

Oedema may cause partial closure of the eye (**Figure 11.3**), but there should be no pain on eye movements and no visual defect.

### Orbital cellulitis

Orbital cellulitis is a relatively rare but serious infection of the tissues behind the orbital septum. It can occur as a complication of the more common preorbital (preseptal) cellulitis. The most commonly implicated organisms are *Staphylococcus aureus* and streptococci.

***Clinical features*** Like preorbital cellulitis, orbital cellulitis can present with erythema, swelling and tenderness of the tissues around the eye. Additional features include:
- proptosis (anterior bulging of the eye)
- pain or limitation on movement of the eye, caused by inflammation of the extraocular muscles
- reduced visual acuity or loss of vision

CT of the orbits should be requested and urgent opinions sought from both the ophthalmology and ENT teams in case surgical drainage is required. Intracranial complications, for example cavernous sinus thrombosis, can occur.

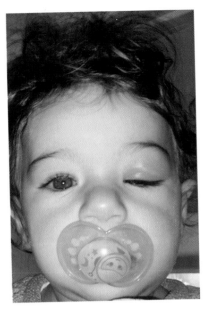

**Figure 11.3** Periorbital cellulitis.

## Painful ear

The differential diagnosis of a painful ear in a child includes:

- foreign body
- acute otitis media
- otitis externa
- mastoiditis
- otitis media with effusion

### Acute otitis media

Acute otitis media is a viral or bacterial infection of the structures of the middle ear. The tympanic membrane is inflamed.

*Clinical features* The most common presentation in a pre-school child is fever and vomiting rather than localising pain. Children may be 'off their food' (through jaw pain), tug at their ear or fall more easily (from dizziness caused by fluid in the middle ear).

Children with Down's syndrome (see page 287) and ciliary dyskinesias are particularly predisposed to ear infections.

## Otitis externa

In otitis externa, there is inflammation of the pinna (the outer ear and earlobe). The causative bacteria include *Pseudomonas* spp., and bacterial swabs should be taken before treatment is commenced.

***Clinical features*** The pinna may appear red, oedematous and crusty. The ear canal may be swollen or completely closed.

## Mastoiditis

Mastoiditis is a local osteomyelitis of the mastoid process, where the sternomastoid muscle attaches to the skull. It is associated with serious complications such as meningitis and venous thrombosis.

***Clinical features*** The first sign of mastoiditis is often the affected ear being pushed forwards by the inflammation behind it (**Figure 11.4**). The mastoid process is tender and red. CT confirms the diagnosis. Intravenous antibiotics are required, as well as urgent referral to ENT surgeons for possible drainage.

## Otitis media with effusion

In otitis media with effusion, there are chronic serous thick secretions behind the eardrum but no acute infection.

***Clinical features*** Children with chronic serous otitis media may develop hearing and speech problems, caused by a conductive hearing defect across the fluid-filled middle ear. Recurrent infections may also occur. Most cases settle spontaneously. If hearing is affected, grommets (small aerating tubes) may be inserted into the tympanic membranes.

## Sore throat

Sore throat is the most common paediatric presentation and involves pharyngitis or tonsillitis. Fever may be the only early presenting sign.

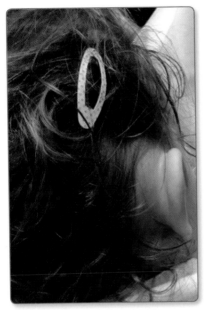

**Figure 11.4** Mastoiditis pushing the pinna forwards.

## Tonsillitis

Tonsillitis has a viral or bacterial cause. It is often difficult to distinguish between the two aetiologies.

*Clinical features*  The hallmark symptoms of tonsillitis are:
- fever
- being 'off food' (because swallowing hurts)
- vomiting

The tonsils are red and often swollen. There may be exudate, pus or even bleeding (**Figure 11.5**). Associated symptoms include:
- cough or coryza (a runny nose) in viral upper respiratory tract infections
- snoring or obstructive sleep apnoea (see page 265) if the tonsils are significantly enlarged

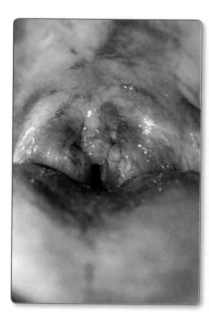

**Figure 11.5** Enlarged tonsils with some bleeding, caused by viral infection.

- lymphadenopathy and petechiae of the palate in glandular fever (Epstein–Barr virus)
- sandpaper rash, red lips and prominent tongue papillae ('strawberry' tongue) in scarlet fever (caused by *Streptococcus pyogenes*)

**Clinical insight**

Do not overlook a history of a recent sore throat. Many autoimmune conditions develop after streptococcal infection. These include rheumatic fever (see page 192), glomerulonephritis and erythema nodosum (see page 253).

## Quinsy

Infection that seeds behind the tonsil causes a peritonsillar abscess or 'quinsy' (**Figure 11.6**). This creates the unusual symptom of unilateral sore throat and requires incision, drainage and antibiotics.

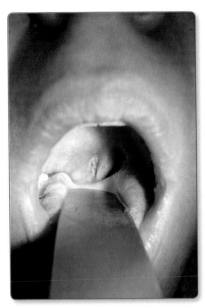

**Figure 11.6** Peritonsillar abscess ('quinsy'). Note the deviation of the uvula.

## Epistaxis

The differential diagnosis of epistaxis includes:

- mucosal trauma
- systemic coagulopathy
- a foreign body in the nose

**Mucosal trauma**  Objects or exploratory fingers that disrupt the thin, highly vascular nasal mucosa can cause bleeding. If the mucosa becomes thinned or swollen during a cold or rhinitis, it becomes more prone to bleeding.

*Clinical features*  Nosebleeds are usually self-limiting. However, the amount of blood often looks impressive because the nose has a large blood supply. Parents should encourage the child to sit with the head held forward and squeeze the soft tissue of the middle of the nose firmly until the bleeding stops.

**Systemic coagulopathy** Bleeding may be prolonged in a child who has an impaired blood clotting cascade. Such conditions are inherited (e.g. haemophilia) or acquired (e.g. idiopathic thrombocytopenic purpura or leukaemia – see pages 250–255).

*Clinical features* Coagulopathies rarely present with a nose-bleed as the sole symptom: there may also be a history of lethargy, easy bruising and bone or joint pain. When a child with a known coagulopathy presents with a nosebleed, a haematologist should be informed and local policies followed.

**Foreign body in the nose** Parents are not always aware that their child has put a small object into his or her nose. This is a common cause of mucosal trauma.

*Clinical features* There may be no obvious sign that something is in the nose, or there may be a small amount of bleeding. If an organic object has been in the nose for a few days, offensive secretions from decomposition may leak from the nose and be noticed by the parents.

### Clinical insight

One method of removing a foreign body is to occlude the unaffected nostril and ask the parent to seal their lips against the child's lips and blow hard; this often causes the object to shoot out of the nose. Foreign bodies can be removed with a probe or suction, requiring a general anaesthetic, if the object is firmly lodged.

## Lumps in the neck

The most common cause of neck lumps in children is lymphadenopathy, which is acute (<2 weeks) or chronic (>2 weeks). Thyroid disease is another cause of a neck mass, and in this case the mass is located in the anterior, not lateral, region of the neck.

### Lymphadenopathy

Lymph nodes are found all over the body, but are clustered at seven key sites. They may be palpable:

- the lateral neck, divided into anterior and posterior triangles (**Table 11.1**)
- behind and in front of the ears
- under the chin
- in the axillae

| Anterior triangle of the neck | Posterior triangle of the neck |
|---|---|
| Anterior cervical lymphadenopathy Submandibular lymphadenopathy Submandibular gland or cyst Thyroid cyst, thyroid mass or diffuse enlargement of the thyroid gland Thyroglossal cyst Parathyroid cyst or mass Skin or subcutaneous tissue lump (e.g. lipoma, sebaceous cyst) | Posterior cervical lymphadenopathy Sternocleidomastoid tumour Cystic hygroma Skin or subcutaneous tissue lump (e.g. lipoma or sebaceous cyst) |

Table 11.1 Differential diagnosis of a neck lump, based on anatomical location

- in the groin
They may also be enlarged:
- at the hilum of the lung, visible on chest radiograph
- at the terminal ileum, causing extreme appendicitis-like pain
Lymphadenopathy is therefore local or systemic, based on whether one or more sites are involved.

The most common causes of lymph node enlargement (**Figure 11.7**) are:
- infection
- malignancy
- autoimmune disease

**Infectious lymphadenopathy** Systemic infection, for example influenza, can cause widespread lymphadenopathy. However, lymph nodes themselves sometimes become infected, as in bacterial lymphadenitis. When lymphadenopathy occurs in the context of a reaction to a local infection elsewhere, the lymphadenopathy is referred to as reactive.

*Clinical features* Reactive lymphadenopathy is usually acute and associated with the symptoms of another infection, for example a sore throat. The affected nodes are often tender and mobile, and there may be overlying erythema. Certain infections (e.g. Epstein–Barr virus, HIV or mycobacteria) also cause chronic lymphadenopathy.

Lymphadenitis may result in a localised abscess, which may need incision and drainage.

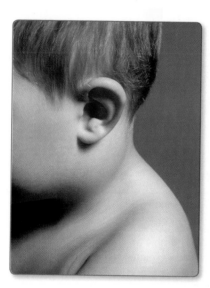

**Figure 11.7**
Lymphadenopathy. This child has enlarged lymph nodes from Epstein–Barr virus infection.

**Malignant lymphadenopathy**  The most common malignancies in children are leukaemia and lymphoma; both cause lymphadenopathy.

*Clinical features*  Malignant lymphadenopathy is usually chronic (>2 weeks' duration). It is either systemic or localised: children with lymphoma classically have localised neck lymphadenopathy. This comprises a group of fixed, matted nodes that are painless and feel firm and rubbery on palpation. There may also be systemic features of the malignancy, such as anaemia, bruising, weight loss and night sweats.

### Thyroid disease

The thyroid gland is situated in the anterior triangles of the neck. It sits in front of and to either side of the trachea and inferior to the cricoid cartilage. In children, the most common cause of diffuse thyroid enlargement or 'goitre' (**Figure 11.8**) is Graves' disease – an autoimmune condition that results in hyperthyroidism.

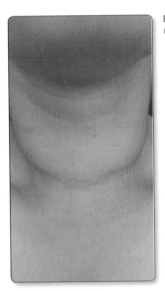

**Figure 11.8** A goitre in a child with Grave's disease.

| Hypothyroidism | Hyperthyroidism |
|---|---|
| Weight gain | Weight loss |
| Slow movements | Hyperactiveness, tremor, jitteriness |
| Slow pulse | Rapid pulse, arrhythmia |
| Slow relaxing reflexes | Hyperreflexia |
| 'Toad-like' facies | Exophthalmos, proptosis |
| Pallor | Flushed or sweaty palms |
| Poor feeding (babies) | Poor feeding (babies) |

**Table 11.2** Symptoms of thyroid disease

*Clinical features*  Either a thyroid nodule is felt within the thyroid, or the thyroid gland is diffusely enlarged. The key feature is a midline swelling that moves with swallowing. Signs and symptoms of thyroid disease are listed in **Table 11.2**, but many goitres are asymptomatic.

# 11.3 Examination of the head and neck

A general ENT examination, including examination of neck masses, proceeds as follows:

- general inspection
- neck examination
- ear examination
- nose examination
- oropharynx examination

## General inspection
### Exposure

Children of all ages can be examined clothed as long as the neck is fully exposed. The ears, nose and throat of younger children are easiest to examine with the child on a parent's knee, as the child generally resists examination.

### General assessment

Inspect for:

- dysmorphia
- facial swelling
- respiratory distress
- scars suggestive of previous surgery (**Figure 11.9**)
- masses and overlying skin colour
- tracheostomy (**Figure 11.10**)
- hearing aids or cochlear implant (**Figure 11.11**)

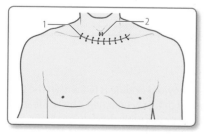

**Figure 11.9** Midline neck scars from ① tracheostomy, and ② thyroidectomy.

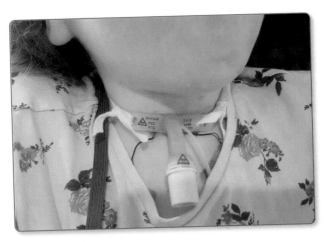

**Figure 11.10** Tracheostomy.

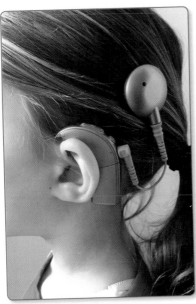

**Figure 11.11** Cochlear implant.

## Neck examination

The neck should be examined as follows:

- inspection
- active movements
- swallowing
- palpation
- auscultation

### Positioning

The child should be inspected from the front, to best visualise asymmetry. Palpation, however, is usually best done from behind (**Figure 11.12**). This can be frightening for younger children so adapt your approach to the compliance of the child; for younger children, it can easily be turned into a tickling game.

### Inspection

Examine the neck for scars or neck masses. Look particularly for goitre (see **Figure 11.8**) and lymphadenopathy (see **Figure 11.7**). Note the colour of the overlying skin.

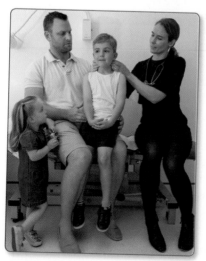

**Figure 11.12** Optimal position for palpating the neck.

## Active movements

Look for restriction of neck movement caused by pain or swelling. Using instruction or distracting toys, get the child to:

- touch their chin to their chest
- touch their ear to their shoulder
- turn their head in each direction
- open their mouth wide
- stick out their tongue (a thyroglossal cyst moves up as the tongue is stuck out)
- reach up to the ceiling and hold the position (an enlarged thyroid will obstruct venous return from the head and the face will become suffused – Pemberton's sign)

## Swallowing

Watch the child swallow a glass of water. A thyroid or parathyroid mass moves with swallowing. Masses in muscle or lymph nodes do not move.

## Palpation

From behind, palpate the thyroid gland if you can. Check that the gland moves with swallowing.

Palpate for lymph nodes:

- in the anterior cervical chain
- in the posterior cervical chain
- under the jaw
- behind the ears
- in front of the ears
- the occiput

Note in particular the:

- texture – fluctuant, firm or rubbery
- contour – smooth or craggy
- mobility – tethered or mobile
- pain – tender or non-tender
- heat – warm to the touch or normal

## Auscultation

Listen over neck masses for bruits. Vascular malformations sound like a heart murmur.

## Ear examination
### Positioning
After looking face-on at the child for signs of asymmetry, get the child to sit sideways across the parent's legs (**Figure 11.13**). Ask the parent to wrap one arm around the child's trunk and arm, and place the other hand on the child's temporal bone, stablising the child's head against the parent's shoulder. This leaves you free to hold the pinna of the child's ear. If the process is gentle and the parent is calm and reassuring, the child should be reassured.

### Inspection
For each ear, examine:
- the pinna, for signs of inflammation, crusting or discharge
- behind the pinna, for inflammation, suggestive of mastoiditis
- the inside of the ear canal, using an otoscope

When using an otoscope, pull the pinna gently backwards (towards the occiput) to straighten the ear canal. Note particularly:
- pus or debris
- foreign bodies
- wax

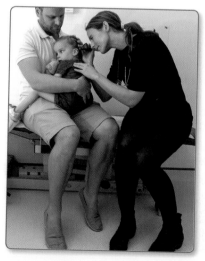

**Figure 11.13** Optimal position for examining the ears.

- the colour of the eardrum
- a fluid level behind the eardrum, suggestive of otitis media
- the contour of the drum (a bulging drum also suggests otitis media)
- a light reflex (a reflection of light from the centre of the eardrum); an absent light reflex is suggestive of fluid in the middle ear

Hearing tests, whether part of a routine screen or where there are concerns about hearing loss, should be formally carried out by an audiologist.

## Nose examination
### Positioning

In younger children, examination of the nose is often best performed with the child initially on the parent's lap.

> ## Clinical insight
>
> Nose picking can cause scratches on the nasal mucosa which will self-resolve without treatment. A septal haematoma, however, is a surgical emergency and requires immediate ENT referral to prevent avascular necrosis of the septum.

The child should be encouraged first to look forwards and then upwards: this can be achieved with distracting toys or bubbles (**Figure 11.14**).

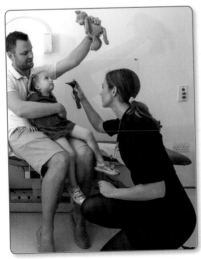

**Figure 11.14** Optimal position for examining the nose.

### Inspection

Inspect the external structures and observe the mucosa over-lying the nasal septum – the septum should be easily visible with a torch. Most children do not tolerate a nasal speculum. The inferior and medial turbinates may be prominent, and can be oedematous in allergic conditions such as rhinitis. Look particularly for foreign bodies.

### Oropharynx examination

Throat examination should be done last in an ENT examination as it is unpleasant for the child.

### Positioning

The child should sit on the parent's lap, with their bottom pushed right back into the parents abdomen. Ask the parent to place one arm across both the child's arms, and the other arm across the child's forehead (**Figure 11.15**). Children often

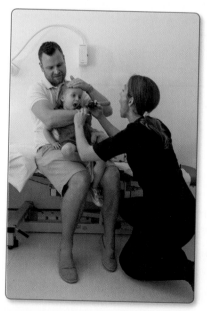

**Figure 11.15** Optimal position for examining the throat.

try to 'slip down' their parent's front but they need to be held upright.

## Inspection

Start with a general examination of the mouth, looking for:

- swelling of the lips
- ulcers
- cold sores
- fetor (bad breath – a sign of tonsillitis)
- the colour of the lips and tongue (especially for pallor or cyanosis)

With a tongue depressor ready, ask the child to say 'aah'. When the child does this, quickly try to get the tongue depressor inside the mouth. Most children will then briefly gag, which, with a light held in your other hand and pointed at the throat, gives a good view of the tonsils and pharynx.

Uncooperative children quickly snap their teeth shut on the wooden tongue depressor. Simply wait patiently; after a while they will open their mouth again to scream or cry, at which point it will be possible to depress the tongue and inspect the pharynx.

Particular areas to examine are the:

- posterior wall of the pharynx, for inflammation in pharyngitis
- palate, for petechiae in Epstein–Barr virus mononucleosis (glandular fever)
- buccal mucosa for ulcers and Koplick's spots (seen in measles)
- uvula for deviation caused by abscess (quinsy)
- general dentition

Inspect the tonsils, on which there may be:

- exudates (pus)
- blood
- multiple small sore vesicular blisters (in herpes simplex tonsillitis)
- unilateral swelling (tonsillar abscess, or 'quinsy')
- a hard yellow/white stone (tonsillolith)

Tonsils are graded using the Brodsky scale according to the proportion of the oropharynx they occlude (**Figure 11.16**). High-grade tonsils are a risk factor for obstructive sleep apnoea (see page 265).

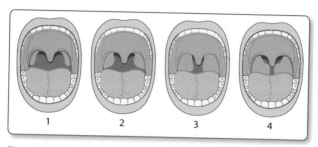

**Figure 11.16** The Brodsky scale of tonsillar size. (1) The tonsils are just visible. (2) The tonsils extend to the tonsillar pillars (<50% of oropharynx). (3) The tonsils cover 50–75% of the oropharynx. (4) The tonsils cover 75–100% of the oropharynx.

## 11.4 Examination summary

A summary of the ENT examination is in **Table 11.3**.

| Component | Key findings |
|---|---|
| General inspection | Weight, height, head circumference, colour, respiratory rate and effort, dysmorphia, masses and swellings |
| Neck | Lymphadenopathy, goitre, swallowing, movements |
| Ears | Swelling, mastoiditis, otitis media, foreign body |
| Nose | Bleeding, haematoma, foreign body |
| Oropharynx | Dentition, fetor, pharyngitis, tonsillitis, quinsy |
| Have you ruled out … ? | Malignancy, foreign body |

**Table 11.3** Summary of the ENT examination

# The skin

Skin is a complicated organ: many diseases manifest as skin lesions, and these are often challenging to describe and analyse. Florid abnormalities are sometimes benign, and small rashes can be a sign of something sinister. Knowing when to worry and when to stay calm is a tricky dilemma for a parent, so rashes are a very common cause of presentation.

This chapter considers not only rashes which are common, but also those which are easily misdiagnosed or mismanaged. The most important rashes to be able to identify are relatively uncommon, but signify severe underlying pathology such as malignancy or sepsis.

## 12.1 Clinical scenario

### Non-blanching rash

A 3-year-old girl is brought to the emergency department by her anxious parents. She recently had a mild cough and cold but has started to develop a rash on her legs and buttocks that does not blanch when pressed with a glass. Her parents are particularly concerned that this is the rash associated with what they call 'meningitis'. The girl is happily playing in the waiting room, and the triage nurse has recorded normal observations.

### Differential diagnosis

This includes:
- benign petechiae relating to vomiting or cough
- meningococcal sepsis
- idiopathic thrombocytopenic purpura (ITP)
- Henoch–Schönlein purpura
- leukaemia

### Further information

The girl looks well and has widespread, slightly raised, purpura on her calves, thighs and buttocks. The purpura is composed of discrete non-blanching areas that have gradually become confluent. There are no petechiae further up the body. There is no pallor or recent weight loss. The systems examination is normal.

## Conclusion

As the child is well, it is very unlikely that this is a presentation of meningococcal sepsis (which many parents call 'meningitis'). The pattern and location of the rash are characteristic of Henoch–Schönlein purpura. However, similarly-presenting serious conditions should be ruled out, for example checking the full blood count and blood film for ITP and leukaemia.

Parents should be reassured that Henoch–Schönlein purpura is often a benign and spontaneously resolving vasculitis that requires no treatment. However, the child should be regularly followed up with urine dipstick and blood pressure checks to rule out renal involvement. The parents should also be told to return to the emergency department if joint or abdominal pains develop.

## 12.2 Common presentations

A rash is any form of inflammation or discoloration that distorts the skin's normal appearance. Types of rash include:

- erythematous
- dry and flaking skin
- urticarial
- maculopapular
- vesicular/bullous
- purpuric/petechial

It is often hard to distinguish similar rashes, for example the maculopapular rashes of scarlet fever, measles and Kawasaki's disease (see page 245), by examination; the history is more useful. This is why the **TENDS** algorithm (see page 5) is so helpful with dermatological conditions. Evolution – where the rash started and how it developed – is often critical to establishing a diagnosis. Examining the child's skin on a single occasion provides only a snapshot of an evolving rash, but regular photographs can be used to stage the progression (see page 253).

Rashes must be distinguished from birthmarks, which are congenital areas of skin discoloration (page 255).

## Erythema

Erythema is redness of the skin, and is one of the four cardinal signs of inflammation (rubor – redness; dolor – pain; tumor – swelling; calor – warmth). Erythematous rashes can be caused by infection, inflammation or contact with skin irritants.

## Cellulitis

Cellulitis is bacterial infection of the dermis (**Figure 12.1**). Underlying structures, such as joints (see page 187) and lymph nodes (see page 225), can also be infected. An infection that tracks along the superficial veins is termed 'phlebitis'.

*Clinical features*  There is a red, hot, spreading patch of painful swollen skin. As well as the joints, infection in the eyelids is particularly worrying (see page 218) as infection can track into the orbit.

**Figure 12.1** Cellulitis.

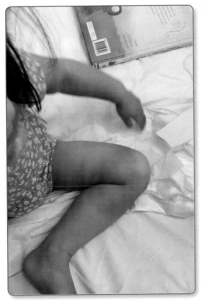

## Nappy rash

Nappy rash (napkin dermatitis) is a painful, red, excoriated rash in the skin creases of children who are not yet toilet trained. Urease enzymes in the faeces convert urea (in urine) into ammonia. This raises the pH of the skin. At this higher-than-normal pH, digestive enzymes in the faeces (proteases and lipases) erode the protective layers of the outer skin, making it more susceptible to irritants in urine, such as urea and ammonia.

## Dry or flaking rashes

In some conditions, a scale may form on top of a rash. Key causes of a scaly or flaking rash include:

- eczema
- psoriasis
- fungal infection
- scabies
- pityriasis rosea

## Eczema

Eczema is the most common skin condition in children. The cause of this inflammation is unknown, although it is strongly associated with atopic conditions, such as asthma and allergies. Eczema can arise anywhere but it most often occurs in flexor areas (the antecubital fossae and popliteal fossae).

*Clinical features* Eczema manifests as local skin dryness, which leads to the development of a scratch–itch cycle. This in turn leads to excoriation and a risk of local infection.

### Clinical insight

Tinea capitis is often misdiagnosed as dandruff or, if a boggy swelling (kerion) is present (**Figure 12.2b**), an abscess.

## Psoriasis

Psoriasis is an inflammatory condition of the skin. The cause is unknown.

*Clinical features* In psoriasis, the skin is thickened and inflamed, with a silvery, scaly appearance. Unlike eczema, psoriasis typically occurs in patches on extensor areas (the elbows and knees). Psoriasis has systemic associations, in particular arthritis. The nail beds may also be involved.

## Fungal infection

Fungal infection presents as raised flaking lesions of the skin
(**Figure 12.2a** and **Table 12.1**).

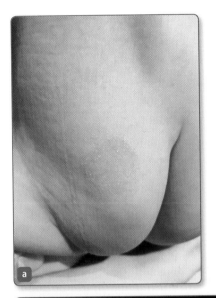

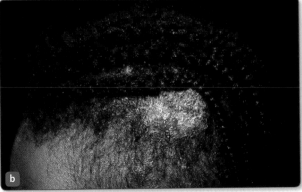

**Figure 12.2** (a) The well-demarcated flaky round lesion of tinea corporis.
(b) Tinea capitis causing a boggy swelling called a kerion.

| Diagnosis | Site | Description |
|---|---|---|
| Tinea capitis | Scalp | Localised area of hair loss or alopecia, with a scaly border |
| Tinea pedis | Foot | Itchy flaking skin between the toes |
| Tinea cruris | Groin | Itchy flaking skin in the groins, skin folds and natal cleft |
| Tinea corporis | Any area | Red, itchy, scaly circular lesion |
| Tinea versicolor | Any area | Small circular areas of depigmentation |
| Candidiasis | Groin, mouth, nipples | White patches on erythematous painful mucosa |

Table 12.1 Fungal infections of the skin

## Scabies

Scabies is a contagious itchy skin infestation caused by the mite *Sarcoptes scabiei*. It is known as 'the seven year itch'.

*Clinical features*  In scabies, the mites tunnel into the skin, particularly through the webbing between fingers, visible as tracking pink trails. The rash is papular and often scabbed from repeated scratching. The hands and wrists are disproportionately affected, but the chest and groin may also be sites of infestation.

## Pityriasis rosea

The cause of pityriasis rosea is unknown, but is possibly a viral infection.

*Clinical features*  The rash is in a 'Christmas tree' distribution (**Figure 12.3**). It usually starts as a single oval 'herald patch' on the trunk, which is often mistaken for a fungal infection because of its shape and texture.

## Urticaria

Urticaria results from the degranulation of histamine by mast cells in the skin. Most cases are idiopathic, but common causes are viral infection and allergy.

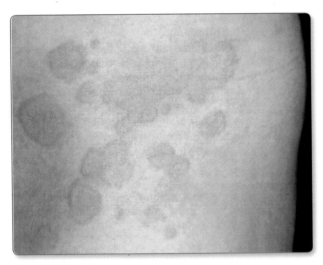

**Figure 12.3** Pityriasis rosea.

*Clinical features* There is a pink, poorly demarcated rash, with discrete, raised, pale, circular lesions ('hives'; **Figure 12.4**). It is usually very itchy.

> **Clinical insight**
>
> Although a simple urticarial rash in adults is usually a sign of allergy, in children <8 years of age it is more commonly a sign of viral infection or is idiopathic. The clue is in the history.

### Erythematous maculopapular lesions

Many rashes are a combination of three appearances: 'erythema' (redness), 'macules' (flat lesions) and 'papules' (raised spots) (**Figure 12.5**).

Examples include:
- viral exanthems, e.g. measles
- Kawasaki's disease
- scarlet fever
- Lyme disease

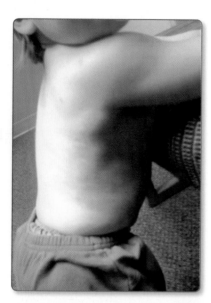

**Figure 12.4** Acute urticaria.

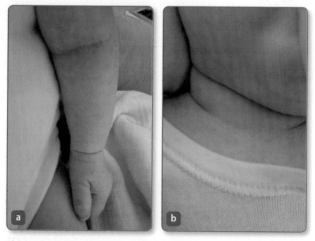

**Figure 12.5** A baby with a maculopapular rash.

## Measles

Measles is a systemic infection caused by a paramyxovirus. It remains one of the main causes of childhood mortality in the developing world. It is preventable with immunisation. In rare cases, it lies dormant in the brain and reappears as subacute sclerosing panencephalitis.

*Clinical features* The rash has a characteristic progression: it starts behind the ears and spreads down the face and across the trunk and back (**Figure 12.6**). It is accompanied by high fevers. The child is miserable, with red conjunctivae. Early in the illness, Koplick's spots (pale blue-white spots) can be seen inside the mouth next to the teeth.

## Kawasaki's disease

Kawasaki's disease is a medium and small vessel vasculitis. The cause is unknown.

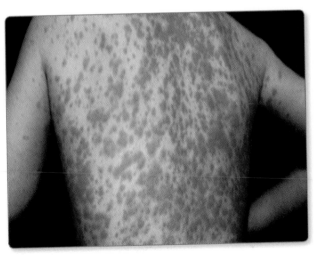

**Figure 12.6** A child with measles.

*Clinical features* In addition to a maculopapular rash (**Figure 12.7**), there is:
- fever continuing for >5 days
- cervical lymphadenopathy
- bilateral non-purulent conjunctivitis
- redness or cracking of the lips
- red and swollen peripheries with peeling skin (a late sign)

Early diagnosis and treatment is crucial to prevent coronary artery aneurysms. All children with suspected Kawasaki's disease should undergo echocardiography.

## Scarlet fever

Scarlet fever is the result of infection with group A *Streptococcus*. Complications include glomerulonephritis and rheumatic fever. It is a notifiable disease in the UK.

*Clinical features* Scarlet fever presents as a classic erythematous maculopapular rash with a sandpaper texture, and often spares the perioral region. Other signs include:
- high fevers
- 'strawberry' tongue with raised papillae
- tonsillitis
- lymphadenopathy

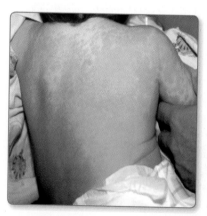

**Figure 12.7** This rash in a febrile child with Kawasaki's disease is also suggestive of measles or scarlet fever. Other diagnostic criteria are required from the history.

- confluent axillary petechiae (non-blanching spots in lines – Pastia's lines)

## Lyme disease

Lyme disease results from being bitten by a tick harbouring the bacterium *Borrelia burgdorferi*.

***Clinical features*** The 'target lesion' (erythema chronicum migrans) is a classic early manifestation of Lyme disease. It has a 'bull's eye' appearance (**Figure 12.8**). If untreated, Lyme disease can cause arthritis, cognitive decline and neuropathy which may manifest months to years after the initial bite.

## Vesicobullous lesions

Vesicobullous lesions are rashes made up of blisters: 'vesiculo' refers to blisters <1 cm wide, and 'bullous' to those >1 cm. Key causes include:
- chickenpox and shingles
- eczema herpeticum
- hand, foot and mouth disease
- molluscum contagiosum
- bullous impetigo
- Stevens–Johnson syndrome

## Chickenpox

Chickenpox is the result of a systemic infection with varicella zoster virus. The virus lies dormant in the dorsal root ganglia of the spine, and spontaneous reactivation can occur without warning or as a result of immunosuppression. This is 'shingles'.

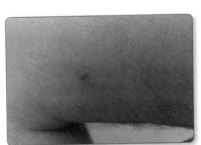

**Figure 12.8** Target lesion of Lyme disease. Note the central punctum from the tick bite, with annular spreading erythema chronicum migrans.

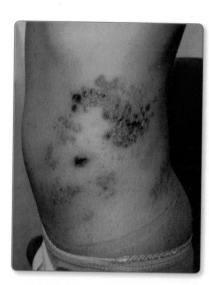

**Figure 12.9** Shingles. Note the dermatomal pattern.

***Clinical features*** Chickenpox initially presents with fever and coryzal symptoms. The rash develops as small, erythematous macules. These form into small blisters (vesicles), rupture and then crust over. The rash may also involve the oral mucosa, which makes drinking very painful. In rare cases, the infection can cause cerebellitis, leading to ataxia (see page 156).

The rash of varicella zoster virus reactivation shingles (**Figure 12.9**) has a classic dermatomal distribution, appearing across the area of skin innervated by one or more adjacent nerve roots.

### Eczema herpeticum

In eczema herpeticum, the thickened, dry and cracked skin of eczema becomes infected with herpes simplex virus (**Figure 12.10**).

***Clinical features*** The affected area of eczematous skin becomes more inflamed, weeps and is covered in small blisters. Herpetic lesions spread quickly to other patches of eczema around the body. Bacterial superinfection is common.

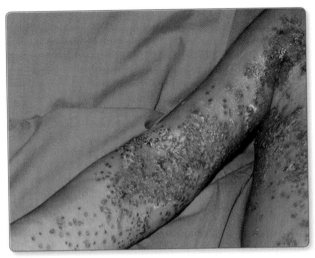

**Figure 12.10** Eczema herpeticum on the arm. Note that the worst disease is found in the flexor creases. Some of the lesions have a golden appearance, which looks like impetigo; this suggests a staphylococcal infection in addition to the herpes simplex virus infection.

## Hand, foot and mouth disease

Hand, foot and mouth disease is caused by a variety of viruses, particularly Coxsackie viruses. It is not related to foot and mouth disease of animals, which parents are often worried about.

*Clinical features* Hand, foot and mouth disease starts with a coryzal illness, often with fever. A papular and then vesicular rash develops in a characteristic distribution. Unlike most viral rashes, it particularly affects perioral and glabrous skin (the palms of the hands and soles of the feet). It requires no treatment.

## Molluscum contagiosum

Despite its name, molluscum is caused by a pox virus and not a parasite.

*Clinical features*  Characteristic pearlescent vesicles appear in discrete areas of skin. These vesicles are filled with clear fluid and have a dipped 'Werther's Original' shape. The rash spreads very easily to previously uninfected areas of skin and can take 18 months to disappear completely. Small scars sometimes form when the vesicles burst.

### Bullous impetigo

Impetigo is an infection of the dermis caused by *Staphylococcus aureus*. Fluid emanating from the infected site can raise a thin-roofed blister (a bulla – **Figure 12.11a**). If these rupture, they leave tender weeping sores (**Figure 12.11b**).

### Stevens–Johnson syndrome

Stevens–Johnson syndrome is usually the result of a drug reaction in which the epidermis and dermis separate. Bullae form on and around the mucous membranes (**Figure 12.12**). In the most severe form, toxic epidermal necrolysis occurs.

### Pupuric/petechial rashes

Purpura describes an area in which blood has extravasated into the skin. Pinprick-sized areas are called petechiae. Just like bruises, these lesions do not blanch on pressure.

The key causes are:
- meningococcal septicaemia
- Henoch–Schönlein purpura
- ITP
- erythema nodosum
- leukaemia

### Meningococcal septicaemia

**Clinical insight**

When a child coughs or vomits forcefully, small blood vessels in the skin may burst and create petechiae. This happens only at or above the level of the superior vena cava.

Bacterial infection of the bloodstream (septicaemia) results in inflammation of small capillary vessels. These vessels become leaky, resulting in intradermal bleeding. Platelet consumption through

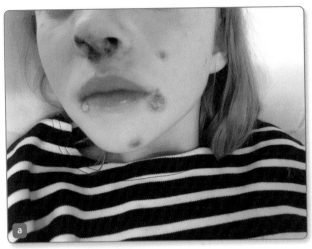

**Figure 12.11** (a) Bullous impetigo. (b) Underlying sore skin when the bullae burst.

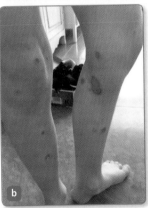

disseminated intravascular coagulopathy compounds this problem.

*Clinical features* A child with meningococcal septicaemia presents as unwell with fevers, limb pain and tachycardia. The level of consciousness may be impaired. Small petechiae initially

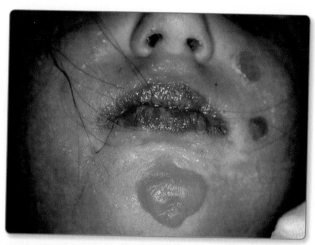

**Figure 12.12** Stevens–Johnson syndrome.

develop and spread, extending in size and forming purpura. The rash evolves quickly (**Figure 12.13**).

## Henoch–Schönlein purpura

Henoch–Schönlein purpura is an idiopathic small vessel vasculitis.

*Clinical features*  The purpuric rash (**Figure 12.14**) occurs mostly over the legs and buttocks, although it also appears on the arms.
The main complications are:

- arthritis, usually affecting large joints, e.g. the knees and ankles
- abdominal pain and, occasionally, intestinal bleeding
- intussusception
- acute glomerulonephritis

## Thrombocytopenic purpura

In ITP, there is an autoimmune consumption of platelets that results in bleeding into the skin. Children present with very low platelet counts ($<10 \times 10^9$/L) but are otherwise systemically well. ITP does not require immediate treatment unless there is

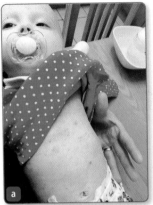

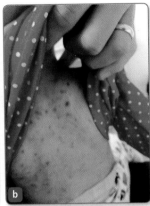

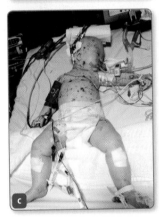

**Figure 12.13** (a) A child 20 minutes after the rash of meningococcal sepsis was identified. (b) The same child 20 minutes later. (c) The same child a little under 12 hours later.

active bleeding or mucosal blistering. However, all children with ITP should be referred to a paediatric haematologist.

### Erythema nodosum

This is a characteristic rash in which painful raised non-blanching lesions are found on both shins. It is caused by inflammation of adipose cells and is associated with a wide spectrum of conditions (**Table 12.2**).

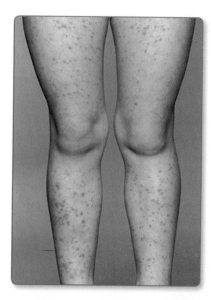

**Figure 12.14** Henoch–Schönlein purpura.

| Category | Examples |
|---|---|
| Autoimmune | Crohn's disease, Behçet's disease, sarcoidosis |
| Infection | *Streptococcus*, *Mycoplasma*, tuberculosis, *Yersinia*, cat scratch fever, Epstein–Barr virus |
| Oestrogen | Oral contraceptive pill, pregnancy |
| Medication reaction | Oral contraceptive pill, penicillins, sulfonamides |
| Malignancy | Non-Hodgkin's lymphoma |
| Idiopathic | The majority – 50% |

**Table 12.2** Causes of erythema nodosum

### Leukaemia

In rare cases, purpura and petechiae are caused by malignancy of bone marrow as the proliferation of lymphoblasts or myelocytes suppresses platelet production. There is usually concomitant anaemia and a significant leucocytosis. Therefore perform

| Birthmark | Description | Action required |
|---|---|---|
| Port-wine stain | Purple, flat, discrete, large, irregularly shaped | If in distribution of CN Va, refer urgently for MRI and ophthalmology assessment to rule out intracranial arteriovenous malformation and glaucoma (Sturge–Weber syndrome) |
| 'Stork' mark | Pink shape on nape of neck, flat, discrete, irregular | None |
| Strawberry naevus | Raised red benign haemangioma, grows and then atrophies over 3–7 years | If >1, or bleeding or growing into eye or airway, refer to dermatology department and arrange US of the abdomen to rule out intravisceral haemangiomas |
| Café-au-lait macule | Oval or irregular, light brown flat macules | If >4 macules, refer to dermatology and genetics departments for possible neurofibromatosis |
| Blue spot | Dark blue discoloration of buttock and sacrum | None |
| CN, cranial nerve. | | |

**Table 12.3** Common birthmarks

a full blood count and film in all children with an unexplained non-blanching rash.

### Birthmarks
Birthmarks are areas of abnormally coloured skin that have been present since the first few days of life. Birthmarks do change in size and shape with time, so it is important to warn parents about their evolution to avoid future distress. Most birthmarks are benign, but multiple marks, or marks in certain locations may be a sign of underlying pathology (**Table 12.3**).

## 12.3 Examination of the skin

A systematic approach to dermatological examination is challenging because so much depends on inspection, and so little on other skills such as auscultation. However, it is possible to break down the examination of the skin into separate sections so that key findings are not missed.

The approach should cover:

- general inspection
- focused description of lesions
- palpation
- examination of commonly overlooked areas

## General inspection

First form a general impression of the child. Do they appear:

- miserable or comfortable?
- scratching or holding part of their body in pain?
- tachypnoeic, febrile or tachycardic?
- lethargic?
- pale?
- dehydrated?

The appearance may suggest sepsis, malignancy or vasculitis.

Plot the height and weight on a growth chart. Chronic conditions such as eczema correlate with reduced growth velocity.

Expose the patient's skin as much as possible. This can be done all in one go with babies and younger children. However, older children tend to prefer a stepwise approach, uncovering and re-covering each limb and body area separately. Always have a chaperone present when exposing groin and breast areas.

Consider whether the underlying skin appears moist or dry. Skin that is dry and flaking may reflect dehydration, eczema or rarer conditions such as ichthyosis (literally 'fish-disease'), in which the skin is scaly.

The bed or the clothing may be stained from bleeding or exudate. Severely eczematous skin sloughs, and there may be dead skin flakes on clothing or furniture.

## Focused description of lesions

You should know the key terms used to describe a rash, and have a structure you can use to depict each property of a lesion or lesions. Rashes and lesions should be described according to:

- distribution
- colour
- size
- shape and pattern

## Distribution of lesions

Examine the whole body and plot the affected areas on a body map to estimate the percentage of body surface area affected. This is especially important when mapping burns if more than 10% of the skin has blistered, life-threatening fluid loss can occur.

Note whether the distribution is:

- dermatomal, as in shingles
- linear, e.g. track marks in the finger and toe web spaces in scabies
- isolated to flexor or extensor areas
- well circumscribed or diffuse
- multiple separate areas or confluent

### Clinical insight

Does the itchy rash spare areas of the back that the patient cannot reach? Impetigo and fungal infections are often spread by scratching.

### Clinical insight

When assessing the distribution of a rash, consider how it relates to clothing. Rashes found only in unclothed areas are likely to be photosensitive in nature. Rashes that occur only where clothes are in contact with the skin may be soap-powder contact dermatitis.

## Colour

Consider the colour of the rash. It may be:

- white, indicating depigmentation – seen in tinea versicolor
- erythematous – seen with many inflammatory rashes and in eczema, measles and Kawasaki's disease
- dark red or blue – seen in vasculitic conditions, e.g. Henoch–Schönlein purpura
- brown – seen in skin lesions that arise from melanocytes, e.g. giant congenital melanocytic naevus
- crusted with yellow or white on top of a different underlying colour, e.g. in erythema – blue, green or yellow of a bruise
- filled with clear or turbid fluid

## Size

Measure the diameter of well-circumscribed lesions or patches.
Fluid-filled lesions are classified according to their individual size:

- vesicular (<1 cm in diameter) – seen in varicella zoster and herpes simplex
- bullous (>1 cm in diameter) – seen in bullous impetigo and Stevens–Johnson syndrome

## Shape and pattern

Lesions may be described as being:

- round
- irregular at the edges
- linear or migrating (e.g. in shingles or cutaneous larva migrans)
- target lesions (e.g. in erythema multiforme or Lyme disease)
- well circumscribed (an abrupt border with normal skin, so that it can be easily drawn around)
- confluent (blending into each other)
- poorly circumscribed (gradually blending into normal skin)
- in the shape of an implement (linear bruises raise the possibility of physical abuse with a belt or cane)

## Palpation

Palpation is an underappreciated aspect of the dermatological examination. Palpate affected areas both gently (to assess texture and tenderness) and firmly (to assess depth and fluctuance).

Lesions may be raised or flat, or a mixture of both. Descriptions that are used to describe the texture of lesions include:

- macular – a flat, non-raised rash
- papular– raised and palpable lesions, seen in acute viral infections and scabies
- scaly – seen in seborrhoeic dermatitis, psoriasis and pityriasis rosea
- crusty – most commonly occurs with exudates, as in impetigo

- fluctuant – fluid-filled lesions may be in the epidermis, like vesicles, or deeper, like abscesses

Be careful not to burst fluid-filled lesions unless you have swabs ready to test for bacterial culture or viral polymerase chain reaction. Bursting lesions can spread infections further.

## Easily overlooked areas

Finally, inspect areas which are easily overlooked:

- scalp – look for hair loss, flaking and rashes hidden in the hair
- neckline – move long hair out of the way to look for non-blanching rashes
- fingernails and toenails – look for pitting, brittle nails and signs of fungal infection
- palms and soles – very few rashes present on glabrous skin

| Component | Key findings |
| --- | --- |
| General inspection | Softness, dryness, icthyosis |
| Lesion distribution | Body mapping, dermatomal distribution, flexure/extensor surfaces, areas spared |
| Lesion colour | Hypopigmentation, bleeding/bruising, erythema, melanocytosis |
| Lesion size and shape | Regularity, irregularity, diameter in centimetres, linearity |
| Lesion contents | Pus, clear fluid, blood |
| Palpation | Texture, tenderness, itching |
| Mucosa | Oral blistering, 'strawberry' tongue |
| Scalp and neck | Flaking, redness, itching, kerions |
| Nails | Pitting, flaking, fungal infection |
| Glabrous skin | Hand, foot and mouth |
| Groin and buttocks | Nappy area, skin creases |
| Have you ruled out … ? | Non-accidental injury, leukaemia, treatable infection |

**Table 12.4** Summary of the paediatric dermatological examination

- tongue and buccal mucosa – raised papillae create the so-called 'strawberry' tongue
- groin and buttocks – look especially for nappy rash and genital inflammation (vulvovaginitis or balanitis)
- breasts – non-blanching rashes may present under bra straps

## 12.4 Examination summary

The skin examination is summarised in **Table 12.4**.

# Abnormal behaviour

Behaviour, more than any physical parameter, alters radically between birth and adulthood. The seemingly random cries and cycles of sleep in neonates evolve into meaningful calls, intended actions and mobilisation within a year (see **Chapter 5**). As children develop, so do their attitudes, interests and personalities.

As they age, children learn different social and emotional skills. It is not possible (or indeed rational) to plead for compassion from a mid-tantrum toddler. Some parents feel the same way about their teenage children as they go through puberty. The under-5s rarely lie, but their experience of truth and unreality are very different from adults', and they are able to engage in incredibly intricate pretend play.

## Reasons for presenting

Behavioural presentations are not uncommon, because parents can be significantly distressed when their children interact socially in an unusual manner. Stigmas are attached to some behavioural diagnoses, and some parents actively resist a diagnosis, unhappy that their child is being labelled as abnormal. Other parents, however, actively seek a diagnosis of, for example, autism spectrum disorder (see page 270) or attention deficit hyperactivity disorder (ADHD; see page 269) because this enables the child to have extra educational support.

Social circumstances and 'life events' also have a significant impact on behaviour. Family fracture, bereavement, friendship and grooming all severely affect behaviour. However, even small everyday aspects of social history, such as diet, hours of television watched and lack of behavioural boundaries, can have surprising influence. Many unusual or difficult behaviours are completely normal, and this can be a challenging conclusion to give to an exasperated parent.

## Parenting

Some parents struggle to control the normal extremes of a child's behaviour because they lack the right tools, resources or experience. A child who is destructive and hyperactive at home but has good reports at school may require only a different style of parenting. Courses are available to teach parents methods of reward and chastisement, and age-appropriate activities, to help children with difficult behaviours. Be careful when discussing these: many parents are offended by the mention of 'parenting classes'.

### Clinical insight

Always confirm what the child's behaviour is in a variety of social situations, including school. Although an organic pathology such as asthma may only be triggered in certain locations, a child cannot have 'ADHD only at home'.

Specialist classes are available for parents of children with special educational needs or autism spectrum disorders. These help parents understand the world from their child's perspective and enable them to engage productively with their child.

# 13.1 Clinical scenarios

## Hyperactive child

A 6-year-old boy is referred to the paediatric outpatient department by his GP after a discussion with the school nurse. The main concern is his baseline hyperactivity: he is unable to concentrate for long on an activity, and distracts himself and other pupils by talking and clowning about. He often has to have 'time-out' in the 'naughty corner', where he is frequently found asleep after a couple of minutes. He has many friends who find him entertaining, if at times, annoying. He is sometimes late to school because of early morning headaches that resolve within an hour.

## Differential diagnosis

This includes:

- poor sleep hygiene, perhaps caused by a lack of routine at bedtime or having a television or a computer in the bedroom

- obstructed breathing and sleep apnoea with repeated waking, which may be due to chronic tonsillitis
- coughing at night, which may be due to asthma, gastro-oesophageal reflux, rhinitis or allergy
- a brain tumour, which can cause nocturnal headache that resolves during the day
- attention deficit hyperactivity disorder

## Further information

The boy enjoys playing in the garden when he gets home from school but struggles to sit still for meals. He falls asleep in front of the television at 6.30 p.m., and has to be woken every morning for school. He snores loudly and has woken his parents up with his loud snuffles. He sometimes wakes up gasping or coughing. Sleep is very poor when he has a cold. There are no allergies and he is otherwise well.

The only finding on clinical examination is grade 3 tonsils. There is no neurological impairment.

## Conclusion

The morning headache merits MRI to rule out a brain tumour. However, this boy has obstructive sleep apnoea and also needs to be investigated with an urgent sleep study. This shows multiple dips in oxygen saturations down to 80% and a raised morning $P\text{co}_2$ of 9.6 kPa, which explains the headache. An adenoidectomy and tonsillectomy are curative of his sleep problems and, thereafter, his behavioural problems.

Children may be hyperactive because of ADHD or because of a genetic syndrome (see **Chapter 14**). However, the most common cause of hyperactivity is, paradoxically, tiredness.

## Low mood

A 14-year-old girl presents to the clinic with low mood. She is struggling to summon the energy to engage with activities that she used to enjoy, such as her school orchestra and Scouts. She feels sluggish and miserable all the time but cannot think why, although she soon has mock examinations . She says she has started to get fatter, although she appears to be on the 50th centile for height and weight.

## Differential diagnosis
This includes:
- normal acceptable low mood
- grief/bereavement
- anorexia nervosa
- depression
- anxiety
- dietary insufficiencies
- hypothyroidism

## Further information
The parents and school confirm the girl's story. Her mood has significantly worsened over the last 2 months, during which she has put on more central fat and gone up a trouser size. She is eating well at school and at home; however, she has developed constipation, requiring macrogol stool softeners from her GP. She is upset that she cannot summon the energy to do the things she likes. Her self-esteem is good, although she is concerned that her skin has become oily and spotty.

## Conclusion
This girl has clinical hypothyroidism. A thyroid function test shows a high thyroid-stimulating hormone level and a very low free thyroxine T4 level. Treatment with thyroxine will improve the skin, bowel habit, girth, mood and energy levels.

# 13.2 Common presentations

Children present with issues related to their behaviour if they are not meeting their social milestones appropriately or have regressed in their interaction with people and activities. Such presentations include:
- fatigue
- hyperactivity
- abnormal interaction

- abnormal eating habits
- abnormal continence

## Fatigue

When a child complains of being 'tired' or 'exhausted', study the history carefully. There is a subtle, but important, difference between lethargy and sleepiness. Lethargy is a subjective or objective feeling of low effort that impairs the child's ability to engage in activity. Sleepiness is an inability to stay awake, but this can often be distracted by activity. It is rare for pathologies that cause lethargy also to cause sleepiness.

### Sleepiness

Sleepiness usually derives from poor quality sleep, with reductions in the amount and quality of deep and rapid eye movement (REM) sleep. The most common causes are poor sleep hygiene (**Table 13.1**), eczema and recurrent nocturnal coughing (**Table 13.2**). With obstructive sleep apnoea, a sleep study shows irregular dips in oxygenation. Acute-onset sleepiness with personality change is a 'red flag' for meningoencephalitis.

> ## Clinical insight
>
> The smartphone has significantly changed clinical practice. Ask the parents to take videos of their child's sleep: a good quality video is sometimes enough to rule a diagnosis in or out.

| Habit | Mechanism of sleep impairment |
|---|---|
| Watching bright screens before bed | Impairs release of melatonin |
| Caffeinated and sugary drinks | Stimulant activity |
| Access to mobile phone | Urge to send and check messages |
| Rarely tidied bedroom | Dust and poor air quality |
| Open windows | Environmental light and noise |
| Poor diet and exercise | Disruption of circadian rhythms |

**Table 13.1** Examples of poor sleep hygiene

| Diagnosis | Key findings | Treatment |
|-----------|--------------|-----------|
| Asthma | Atopy, wheeze, worse around smoke or dust | Salbutamol and steroids |
| Posterior nasal drip | Atopy, sneezing, swollen turbinates | Antihistamines and corticosteroid |
| Gastro-oesophageal reflux | Supine chest pain, vomiting, worse after meals | Proton pump inhibitors |
| Obstructive sleep apnoea | Snoring and snuffling, episodes of apnoea and gasping | Adenotonsillectomy, nocturnal continuous positive airway pressure ventilation |
| Tuberculosis | Night sweats, haemoptysis | Quadruple-therapy antibiotics |

**Table 13.2** Differential diagnosis for nocturnal coughing

## Clinical insight

Teenagers may go through periods of withdrawing from their parents, which might be interpreted as social withdrawal. However, a good social history allows you to distinguish between self-isolation in the family home and anhedonia. Children grow out of interests – do not overplay the importance of not enjoying things that formerly were interesting; instead establish whether the child has new interests.

### Lethargy

Rule out organic causes of lethargy (**Table 13.3**) before making a psychiatric diagnosis.

### Depression

Depression affects up to 2% of school-age children and must be carefully distinguished from normal extremes of emotion, such as grief, which can present similarly.

*Clinical features* Depression is a persistent, unremitting feeling of poor self-worth, failure, misery and low energy, which can manifest as social isolation. A key symptom is anhedonia – the inability to enjoy things, including things previously enjoyed. Physical symptoms include appetite change and sleep disturbance. There may be a precipitating life event, a history of bullying or abuse, or a family history of depression.

| Cause | Other symptoms | Risk factors | Test (findings) |
|---|---|---|---|
| Anaemia | Pallor, tachycardia | Heavy periods Vegetarian diet Haemoglobinopathy Helicobacter pylori gastritis | Full blood count (low haemoglobin) |
| Iron deficiency | Alteration of appetite and taste Anaemia | Vegetarian diet Heavy periods Malabsorption | Full blood count (high red cell distribution width*) Iron studies (low serum iron, high iron binding capacity) |
| Vitamin D deficiency | Bone pain Reduced exercise tolerance | Vegan diet Dark skin Low sun exposure Malabsorption (e.g. cystic fibrosis) | Serum vitamin D (low) Bone profile (hypocalcaemia) |
| Hypothyroidism | Weight gain, oily skin, constipation, bradycardia, feeling cold | Autoimmune disease Down's syndrome Family history Goitre | Serum thyroid-stimulating hormone (high) Serum free thyroxine (low) |
| Influenza infection | Fever, myalgia | Unvaccinated | Viral polymerase chain reaction on nasal secretions |
| Post-viral | None | History of significant viral illness | None |

*A high red cell distribution width (RDW) is a much more specific indicator of longstanding iron deficiency than the low mean corpuscular volume (MCV)

Table 13.3  Causes of lethargy

## Chronic fatigue syndrome

Chronic fatigue is poorly understood and is to some degree a diagnosis of exclusion. It presents as idiopathic profound fatigue lasting at least 6 months that impairs simple activities of daily living. The cause is unknown, and treatment is supportive.

## Hyperactivity

Hyperactivity is common in children. It refers to a spectrum of behaviours that includes fidgeting, pacing and inability to sit still. At its extreme, hyperactive children can seem 'always on the go', bouncing around the furniture without regard for safety or other people. Bouts of hyperactivity can occur when children are overexcited, hyperstimulated or 'overtired'. Symptoms are often worse in the family home than at school, where more rigid rules and behavioural restrictions are in place. Some common medications, such as salbutamol, can cause hyperactivity.

A differential diagnosis for persistent hyperactivity includes:
· poor quality sleep (see page 265)
· hyperthyroidism
· anxiety
· ADHD

## Hyperthyroidism

Hyperthyroidism, or 'thyrotoxicosis', is caused by hypersecretion of thyroxine from the thyroid gland. This is usually an autoantibody-mediated process (Graves' disease), but is occasionally caused by increased thyroid-stimulating hormone production by the pituitary gland.

*Clinical features*  Graves' disease frequently presents as a subjective feeling of agitation and is often misdiagnosed as anxiety or panic attacks. Patients feel warm and flushed, and there are often palpitations with tachycardia, and diarrhoea. The heightened metabolic rate causes weight loss and sweating. If it is left untreated, exophthalmos can occur. There may be a goitre.

## Anxiety

Anxiety is a very common symptom and can be normal. For example, infants display separation anxiety – an increase in distress and clinginess when the parent moves away from them – at 8–36 months of age, and this can extend into early school age. Childhood phobias and examination stress are both normal, spontaneously resolving, non-pathological phenomena.

*Clinical features* Pathological anxiety may present acutely as a panic attack. Alternatively, it is sometimes a chronic state of anxiety so hyperacute that it prevents engagement with activity.

Chronic symptoms include difficulty sleeping, bed-wetting and agitation. Children may lose the confidence to try new things or deal with simple everyday activities, such as seeing their friends. Perseveration on possible – sometimes outlandish – negative consequences of simple actions is characteristic. Chronic uncertainty, such as disruptive home life and moving schools, can have a significant negative effect.

## Attention deficit hyperactivity disorder

Attention deficit hyperactivity disorder (ADHD) affects roughly 2% of children, to a varying degree. It can only be diagnosed in children over the age of 6 years because the symptoms and signs are normal behaviours in much younger children and are usually grown out of.

*Clinical features* Great care must be taken in diagnosing ADHD. Its symptoms include very common behaviours such as being easily distracted, forgetfulness, careless mistakes and being unable to stick with time-consuming tasks – all of which may simply be the sign of a bored child. Key symptoms are hyperactivity and impulsiveness, including a lack of awareness of danger and being unable to share in activities or conversation. The symptoms must be permanent and not associated with one particular environment or circumstance.

Always corroborate reports of hyperactivity with information from a child's schoolteacher. A child with ADHD is equally excitable in the home and classroom. A child who is well behaved in maths, art and technology lessons, but whose English teacher worries about ADHD, may be dyslexic and not engaging with one type of lesson.

## Abnormal interaction

All aspects of social interaction, from eye contact to conversational style, alter with age. Atypical social behaviours may be noticed at any age, depending on how severe they are and how well the child masks the symptoms. Some seemingly abnormal behaviours are relatively common and can be grown out of.

Common presentations include:

- breath-holding attacks
- sensory or speech impairment
- depression (see page 266)
- autism spectrum disorder
- anxiety (see page 268)
- genetic syndromes

## Breath-holding attacks

Breath-holding attacks are most common in children aged 8 months to 2 years, although they can occur up to age 5. They occur during tantrums, and are apnoeic episodes during which the child becomes pale or cyanosed and then collapses. Similar to reflex anoxic seizures (see page 114), there is no post-ictal state, and children grow out of this behaviour. The attacks are very frightening to observe but are benign.

## Sensory or speech impairment

Children who cannot see or hear properly may display signs of abnormal social interaction such as ignoring commands (in deafness) or abnormal eye contact (in visual impairment). An isolated speech delay may result in behaviours that are abnormal for the child's age. For example, a 7-year-old who cannot ask to share toys will snatch objects, but does not necessarily lack the social understanding that such behaviour is unacceptable.

## Autism spectrum disorder

Autism spectrum disorder is common, affecting roughly 1% of children, more commonly boys. It is underdiagnosed in both sexes but very significantly so in girls. The spectrum spans a wide range from profoundly disabled non-verbal children to ultra-high-achieving ones.

*Clinical features*  The characteristic features of autism spectrum disorder are social and communication deficits with restrictive, repetitive patterns of behaviour. Examples include:

- poor, unusual or absent eye contact
- difficulty interpreting and using non-verbal communication (facial expression)

- Mind-blindness (inability to see things from another person's perspective (e.g. showing a theory of mind deficit on the Sally–Anne test)
- taking metaphor literally
- difficulty with novelty or unpredictability
- limited pretend play (e.g. sorting cars into colours, not driving them around)
- social isolation
- inability to share
- tantrums when unable to get their own way
- sensory sensitivities
- rigid rules-based patterns of behaviours
- limited obsessive interests (e.g. watching the same video over and over again)
- unusual interests (e.g. car number plates)
- echolalia
- stereotyped movements

Girls with autism spectrum disorders socially isolate themselves less than boys, which makes diagnosis more of a challenge.

### Genetic syndromes

Genetic syndromes present diversely, from social developmental regression (e.g. Rett's syndrome; see page 297) to overfamiliarity (Williams' syndrome; see page 293). These conditions are discussed in **Chapter 14**.

### Abnormal eating habits

Common presentations include:

- fussy eating
- anorexia nervosa
- pica

### Fussy eating

Many children go through a phase of fussy eating. Sometimes, however, they present with pathology that is either the cause or the result of fussy eating (**Table 13.4**).

If not caused by pathology, fussy eating can be managed with non-food rewards and by making mealtimes less antagonistic.

| Cause of fussy eating | Explanation |
|---|---|
| Milk allergy | Pain caused by allergy manifests as feed refusal in babies |
| Gastro-oesophageal reflux | Refusal of food that exacerbates reflux |
| Coeliac disease | Refusal of food that exacerbates pain |
| Meal scheduling problems | Too tired to eat if meals are served late |
| Autism spectrum disorder | Sensitivity to texture, flavour or presentation of food |
| Anorexia nervosa | Anxiety about nutritional content of food |
| Iron deficiency | Alteration of sense of taste |
| **Result of fussy eating** | **Explanation** |
| Failure to thrive/weight loss | Reduced calorie intake |
| Fatigue | Iron and vitamin D deficiencies |
| Social anxiety | Concern that food served in school or with friends will not be tolerable |
| Constipation | Poor fibre intake |
| Obesity | Diet restricted to high-fat or high-sugar foods |

**Table 13.4** Pathologies associated with fussy eating.

## Anorexia nervosa

Anorexia nervosa affects 0.4% of males and 4% of females , the most common age of onset being adolescence. It carries the highest mortality rate of any psychological disorder: over a 10-year-period, the mortality rate is 5%. This is not just from starvation, but includes a suicide risk 56 times the base average.

*Clinical features* Anorexia manifests as a loss of appetite, negative body image, often with a delusory perception of being too fat, and an obsession with weight loss. Individuals with anorexia display significant anxiety about the calorie content of food and try to restrict their diet in an attempt to lose weight.

Societal factors are suggested to play a key role, particularly in children with interests in performing arts and gymnastics. However, life events such as bullying and bereavement are common triggers. There is significant overlap with clinical depression (see page 266).

The diagnosis can only be made in the context of demonstrable weight loss.

## Pica

Pica is the wilful ingestion of non-nutritious matter. Some children eat one particular thing, such as hair (particularly in trichotillomania – compulsive hair plucking). Other children feel compelled to eat almost anything, from foodstuffs to soil. The more severe end of the pica spectrum is associated with severe

### Clinical insight

Children like to put things in their mouths. It is common in emergency department to see children who have swallowed a coin or button battery. Button batteries are corrosive so they must be identified rapidly. They are distinguished from coins on a radiograph by the 'double rim' (Figure 13.1). Button battery ingestion is a surgical emergency because the current generated can erode and perforate tissue structures in as little as 20 minutes.

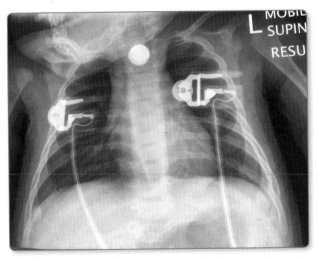

**Figure 13.1** The 'double rim' sign in a baby who was 'fed' a button battery by an older sibling. If a coin had been swallowed, there would be one radio-opaque outline.

learning difficulties and Prader–Willi syndrome (see page 294). Children with pica are at risk of toxin ingestion and developing bezoars (matted lumps of undigestable material that can cause intestinal obstruction).

## Abnormal continence

Children develop urinary and faecal continence over the first 3–4 years of life (see **Chapter 5**). Delays in development of continence and regressions in continence need to be investigated.

The differential diagnosis includes:

- spinal tumour (compression of nerve roots to bowel or bladder; see page 157)
- constipation (compression of bladder neck and overflow diarrhoea; see page 125)
- nocturnal enuresis
- encopresis
- recurrent UTI

### Nocturnal enuresis

It is essential to distinguish the child who has never been dry at night (primary nocturnal enuresis) from the child who has been fully continent for months but has regressed to bed-wetting (secondary nocturnal enuresis).

Primary nocturnal enuresis is surprisingly common and can be present up to the age of 7 years in healthy children. Behavioural techniques such as star charts, toilet training and warning monitors may help; if they do not, medication (desmopressin) can be prescribed.

Secondary nocturnal enuresis is commonly caused by anxiety (see page 268). However, organic pathology such as nocturnal seizures or a spinal tumour may have to be ruled out.

### Encopresis

Encopresis is the soiling of underwear by the passage of faeces. This may be deliberate, habitual or the result of diarrhoeal overflow from constipation (see page 125). Habitual encopresis requires active toilet training and encouragement of regular toilet use (withholding stool at school is a common habit of children). Deliberate soiling may involve smearing faeces around the home and may be a manifestation of a behavioural disorder that requires referral to a psychologist.

# 13.3 Examination of behaviour

Behavioural examination is challenging because there is no 'hands-on' aspect to the process. You cannot palpate or auscultate autism. Instead, the behavioural examination involves a focused history from both child and parent, concentrating on a combination of mental state and social development.

Take as much of the history as possible from the child, and corroborate it with information from the parent. If you talk to the parents first, it can feel like adults 'ganging up' on a child who already feels vulnerable. Information gleaned from both parties during the assessment can be correlated with or called into question by general inspection.

## Environment and ethics

As with the developmental assessment (see **Chapter 5**), the best environment for conducting a behavioural assessment is in a large, colourful room with toys and distractions for younger children. Older children can be assessed in a more formal environment if they prefer.

For teenagers in particular, the behavioural assessment involves talking about very personal issues such as mood, body image, sexual behaviour and suicidal ideation. Teenagers may feel embarrassed opening up about these issues in front of their parents. Therefore it is a good idea to ask the parents to step outside for a few minutes so you can talk to the child on their own, in the company of a chaperone.

Some information the child provides does not need to be passed on to the parents. For example, it is reasonable to talk to a child about their sexuality without informing their relatives. However, in certain circumstances, information will have to be shared with the parents, for example, if the child's safety is at risk, and you should consult a senior colleague before doing so.

## Examination

Taking a stepwise approach to analysing behaviour prevents missing key information. Many professionals, including nurses, schoolteachers, social workers, educational psychologists and care workers, will need information from your assessment. Each will focus on a different part of your assessment to aid their own diagnosis and management.

Use the mnemonic **ASTHMATICS** to remember the behaviours you need to observe and ask about:

- **A**ppearance
- **S**ocial behaviour
- **T**hought content
- **H**unger
- **M**ood
- **A**ffect
- **T**oilet
- **I**nsight
- **C**ognition
- **S**leep

Differentiating benign eccentric, or embarrassing, behaviours from pathological ones is a significant challenge. Many children grow out of unusual behaviours, such as fussy eating or taking the kettle to bed instead of a teddy bear. A thorough **ASTHMATICS** approach elucidates a differential diagnosis, or provides enough structured information to discuss the child in detail with an appropriate specialist.

### Appearance

Observe the child's general appearance and manner:

- Clothing – does the child appear well cared for? Does clothing fit properly or is it baggy? Is it gender-concordant?
- Scars – are there marks of self-harm?
- Interaction – is the child taking part in the consultation, ignoring it or distracted?
- Activity – is the child hyperactive or calm?
- Physical signs – is the child flushed? Are there visible clinical signs such as proptosis or goitre? Does the child have a dysmorphic appearance (see **Chapter 14**)?

## Social behaviour

The content, rhythm and quantity of speech should be noted:

- Is the child speaking to you? Are they naturally shy?
- Is the content monosyllabic or detailed? Is there pressured speech?
- Does the content make sense?
- Are the parents talking for the child, or over the child?
- Does the child understand metaphor?
- If asked to list some animals, does the child have a systematic approach starting with common ones, or do they list unusual ones like ibex and brontosaurus?
- Is their eye contact normal during speech? Is it avoided or uncomfortably persistent?
- Is the tone of voice normal? Exaggerated-timbre 'cocktail party chatter' is characteristic of Williams' syndrome. A robotic nasal timbre devoid of emotional tune occurs in autism spectrum disorders.

Ask about friendships and relationships:

- Do they understand friendships? Do they have any/many good friends?
- Does the child have a boyfriend or girlfriend? Are they sexually active?
- Does the child have people of a very different age whom they think of as friends?
- Does the child behave unusually around other people? Are they anxious, shy or unaware of danger?
- Do they understand facial expressions, body language or social conventions? Does the child behave differently at home from at school?
- Does the child engage in team activities and sharing, or do they isolate themselves?

## Thought content

Assessment of 'thought content' involves discussing persistent and invasive thoughts:

- Does the child have a proportionate understanding of their body image?
- Do they have obsessions – routines, thoughts, interests or behaviours that affect their own or their parents' lives?

- Does the child have an age-appropriate engagement with pretending? Do they play with toys in the same way as their friends? For example, how does the child play with toy cars – by driving them around or by sorting them by colour?
- Does the child hear voices?
- Is there an imaginary friend they speak to?
- What is the child interested in? Do they have a variety of hobbies and interests?

## Hunger

It is important to discuss the child's normal diet. Vitamin and mineral deficiencies can cause profound tiredness and unusual feeding behaviours.

- Does the child have a good appetite?
- Are they careful or fussy about what they eat?
- Are there aversions to certain textures, flavours or colours of food?
- Are they increasingly obsessed with 'healthy' eating or calorie counting?
- Is the child vegan or vegetarian? Is the family?
- Does the child play with or avoid their food?
- Does the child eat unusual things like paper or hair?

## Mood

How does the child feel? Ask about:

- tiredness
- enthusiasm
- self-worth
- suicidal ideation
- potential
- sympathy
- mood swings – does the child have furious outbursts?

## Affect

Affect is the outward portrayal of mood. Does the child look:

- anxious?
- depressed?
- hyperactive?
- eager?

- neutral?
- and does this match their reported mood?

## Toilet

Ask about bowel and bladder function. Constipation, for example, can be a sign of hypothyroidism when coupled with low energy and mood, and may distinguish between an organic and a psychiatric problem in a depressed child. Ask about:

- bowel frequency and stool type
- resistance to using the toilet at school
- bladder frequency and thirst
- bed-wetting
- continence
- deliberate soiling in the home
- cleanliness and handwashing

## Insight

Insight is the patient's understanding of whether their behaviour is normal or irrational. For example, a teenager with a phobia of clowns will know that their fear is irrational but will not be able to repress it. However, a teenager with anorexia nervosa will have a firmly held body image that is very different from the objective reality.

- Does the child feel that their behaviour is a problem?
- Does the child want to change, or want the world around them to change?
- Does the child understand how and why other people react to them?
- Has the child had age-inappropriate experiences that they have normalised, e.g. sexual contact, physical chastisement or emotional abuse?
- Is the child engaged in an activity that they know to be illegal, e.g. under-age drinking and smoking, or drug taking?

## Cognition

Cognition is the ability to process information. Ask about the following:

- Attention – is the child easily distracted, sleepy, or obsessive?

- Logic – are the child's thoughts coherent for their age? Is there knight's move logic (a lack of connected thinking, manifesting as sudden changes of logic and discourse)? Can the child lie?
- Memory – is the child forgetful or unable to learn? Can the child remember unusual things in detail, e.g. car number plates? Does the child have an encyclopaedic memory of certain topics?
- Novelty – does the child react unusually to new situations or information?
- Education – how is the child progressing at school?

## Sleep

Good quality sleep has a huge impact on cognition and behaviour. Ask about the following:
- Is there daytime tiredness and sleepiness?
- Sleep hygiene – note screen time, bedtime, caffeine, high-energy foods and drinks, and exercise.
- Sleep duration – does the child go to bed and struggle to sleep? Or wake early or late?
- Nightmares – is the child distressed at night?
- Enuresis – is there age-inappropriate bed-wetting? Had there been a period of nocturnal continence?
- Noise – does the child snore, cough or gasp during the night?

## Investigations

Depending on the results of the behavioural examination, you may want to consider:
- thyroid function tests, vitamin D and iron status if the child is tired
- an ear, nose and throat examination looking for tonsillar hypertrophy (see **Chapter 11**)
- a sleep study to assess for sleep apnoeas and sleep architecture
- genetic studies if a genetic syndrome is suspected (see **Chapter 14**)
- formal school observation to corroborate (or not) the child's behaviour
- a developmental assessment, with input from the multidisciplinary team (see **Chapter 5**)

- a home visit by a health visitor to assess the family home
- formal referral to a child or adolescent mental health service

## Discussion

The most important part of a behavioural assessment is to establish, using the detailed approach above, whether the child is in danger or is a danger to other people. A violent or suicidal child may need to be admitted to a place of safety while a child psychiatrist undertakes a formal mental health examination. Equally swift intervention is needed if it is suspected that the child is the victim of abuse.

## 13.4 Examination summary

A summary of the behavioural examination is given in **Table 13.5**.

| Component | Key findings |
|---|---|
| Appearance | Dysmorphia, developmental delay, unkemptness, scars |
| Social | Monosyllabic or pressured speech, abnormal speech content, abnormal eye contact, age-inappropriate friends and relationships, mind-blindness22 |
| Thought | Delusions and hallucinations, obsessions and body image, unusual playing or lack of imagination |
| Hunger | Fussy eating, pica |
| Mood | Lethargy, anxiety, outbursts, suicidal ideation |
| Affect | Hyperactivity, social anxiety |
| Toilet | Enuresis, encopresis and continence, hygiene |
| Insight | Unusual beliefs |
| Cognition | Inattention, falling asleep, poor memory or deteriorating schoolwork |
| Sleep | Poor sleep hygiene, coughing, snoring and gasping |
| Have you ruled out … ? | Organic diseases, sensory impairment, child abuse, suicide risk |

**Table 13.5** Summary of the paediatric behavioural assessment

# Genetic disorders and syndromes

## chapter 14

Each of the previous chapters has dealt with an isolated organ system or a particular focused approach to examination. However, all healthcare professionals will find that a significant proportion of their clinical workload relates to a broader set of abnormalities involving multiple systems, especially when working with children. Such cases are syndromes.

Different syndromes present at different stages of life. Some are common and obvious, others more subtle. Owing to their multisystem involvement, it is important to reach a diagnosis as early as possible to prevent complications. Many syndromes can be diagnosed at birth or even during antenatal scanning.

As syndromes present with abnormalities in any organ system, developmental modality or behaviour, all the techniques described in previous chapters are required when examining a child for signs of a genetic syndrome. However, some key skills, for example characterising dysmorphia (unusual facial or bodily structural features), are unique to a syndromic examination.

## Genetic, inherited and congenital

It is easy to misunderstand key terms when discussing syndromes: the terms 'genetic', 'inherited' and 'congenital' are often misused synonymously.

**Genetic conditions** result from an abnormality in the number of chromosomes, or mutations in the nucleotide sequence so have wide-ranging effects; examples include Down's syndrome (see page 287) and cystic fibrosis.

**Inherited conditions** are genetic and have also been passed on from parent to child. Down's syndrome is therefore genetic but not inherited, whereas cystic fibrosis is both genetic and inherited.

**Congenital abnormalities** are present from birth but need not be genetic. For example, toxic damage in utero can cause congenital syndromes that are neither inherited nor genetic; an example is fetal alcohol syndrome (p. 300). Conversely, genetic conditions need not be congenital. For example, Huntington's disease does not manifest until middle age, when symptoms of a neurodegenerative movement disorder start to be seen.

# 14.1 Clinical scenarios

## Short stature

A 10-year-old girl is referred by her GP to the paediatric clinic because of short stature. She was born at term to unrelated parents. She receives annual follow-up for a horseshoe kidney but is taking no medication. Apart from this, she has been generally fit and well. She has always been short, has not yet entered puberty and seems to be falling behind the other girls in her class. Her mid-parental height lies on the 91st centile, but she is growing along the 9th.

### Differential diagnosis

This includes:

- constitutional short stature
- nutritional deficiencies
- neglect
- chronic disease
- growth hormone deficiency
- genetic syndromes
- chondroplasias/dwarfism

### Further information

There is a squat appearance, with a wide neck and shield-shaped chest. The body is in proportion. The Tanner stage is 1 (no breast buds) and there are widely spaced nipples. The fourth finger on each hand is shortened, and a systolic heart murmur is present. The girl is doing adequately academically and has not missed any school days over the last 4 years.

### Conclusion

This girl has the features of Turner's syndrome (page 288), which can be confirmed by karyotyping. If the result is negative, Noonan's syndrome (page 297) should be considered as this has similar features. The heart murmur should be urgently investigated to rule out a coarctation of the aorta or aortic valve abnormality. The diagnosis helps to explain the aetiology of the horseshoe kidney. Pelvic ultrasound should be performed to investigate for streak ovaries, and an endocrinologist will need to determine whether the girl will require medication to enter puberty. Genetics, endocrinology and cardiology specialist referral is necessary.

## Unusual behaviour

A 4-year-old boy is referred to the community paediatrics service by his day nursery as staff are concerned that he might have autism. Particular concerns are his sensory sensitivities to noise, overfamiliarity and peculiar manner of talking. He babbles at people with an exaggerated vocal tone and when asked to name animals will list complex and rare animals. He has very poor motor and visuospatial skills: he cannot skip or draw a circle. The nursery staff are also worried about his dentition.

### Differential diagnosis

The differential diagnosis includes:

- autism spectrum disorder
- idiopathic learning difficulties
- sleep disorders
- genetic syndromes
- non-genetic syndromes
- congenital infections
- neglect

### Further information

The child is socially overfamiliar, makes very strong eye contact and has a cocktail-party style of conversation. It is difficult to engage him in visuospatial tasks. He was quite floppy when he was born and always a little behind with his development. However, while he was waiting for a developmental assessment, he met his milestones so the parents did not attend the appointment.

The boy is well cared for, but there are widely spaced spiked teeth, for which the parents have not sought dental treatment.

A heart murmur is heard in the pulmonary area. He has a wide smile with a flattened nose and long philtrum.

## Conclusion

This child has features of Williams' syndrome, which can be confirmed on genetic testing. An echocardiogram will establish whether there is significant pulmonary stenosis, and a bone profile check will assess whether there is hypercalcaemia.

# 14.2 Common presentations

Common presentations of genetic disorders and syndromes include:
- abnormal antenatal scans
- congenital hypotonia
- abnormal facies (dysmorphia)
- multiple physical abnormalities on a neonatal check
- developmental delay
- family history
- abnormal growth patterns
- common symptom with a genetic basis

These presentations represent syndromes caused by a variety of mechanisms:
- karyotype disorders
- microdeletion syndromes
- autosomal dominant inheritance
- X chromosome linkage
- autosomal recessive inheritance
- non-genetic syndromes

## Karyotype disorders

The karyotype is the complete set of chromosomes in the cell's nucleus. A healthy human karyotype comprises two copies of each of chromosomes 1–22, plus two sex chromosomes (two X chromosomes in girls; one X and one Y chromosome in boys). The normal karyotype is referred to as 46XX (female) and 46XY (male).

A karyotype disorder derives from an incorrect number of chromosomes. The most common examples are:
- Down's syndrome (trisomy 21)

- Edwards' syndrome (trisomy 18)
- Patau's syndrome (trisomy 13)
- Turner's syndrome (XO)
- Kleinfelter's syndrome (XXY)

## Down's syndrome

Down's syndrome is the most common non-idiopathic cause of learning disability and one of the most common genetic disorders.

It arises from excess copies of the genes on chromosome 21, usually pure trisomy (although mosaicism is possible). The unbalanced translocation of a chromosome 21 during meiosis is a chance event that increases in frequency as the mother gets older. For this reason, the probability of conceiving a fetus with Down's syndrome rises with maternal age, from approximately 1:800 at age 30 years to 1:100 at age 40 years.

Down's syndrome is associated with learning difficulties and a characteristic appearance (**Figure 14.1**). Babies with Down's syndrome are often very hypotonic at birth.

Children with Down's syndrome are at increased risk of a number of abnormalities and conditions (**Table 14.1**). They should be screened for these at birth (even leukaemia can be congenital).

The severity of complications varies greatly. It is incorrect to assume that a child with Down's syndrome has multiple medical needs or requires a special school. Some individuals with trisomy 21 are healthy individuals, live independently, hold down long-term jobs and have only mild learning difficulties.

*Clinical features*  These include:

- epicanthic folds
- slanted palpebrae
- low-set ears
- small mouth
- large tongue
- shortened neck
- flat-topped head
- short stature
- single palmar crease
- sandal-gapped toes

### Clinical insight

In Down's syndrome, there is an increased risk of hypothyroidism and leukaemia. Affected children require regular follow-up and annual blood tests to assess thyroid function and blood films. They must also be screened for signs of coeliac disease and sleep apnoea.

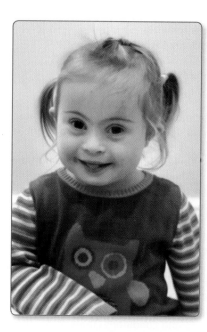

**Figure 14.1** A girl with Down's syndrome. She has low-set ears, slanted palpebrae, a small mouth with a prominent tongue and flat-topped head.

## Edwards' and Patau's syndromes

Other trisomies include trisomy 18 (Edwards' syndrome) and trisomy 13 (Patau's syndrome). Like Down's syndrome, they present with multiple organ involvement and anatomical abnormalities. Unlike Down's syndrome, however, they confer a very poor prognosis, with most children dying in the neonatal period.

The features of Edwards' and Patau's syndromes are listed in **Table 14.2**.

## Turner's syndrome

Turner's syndrome (45XO) occurs where there is absence of one X chromosome in a person who is phenotypically female. About 1% of all in utero fertilisations have a Turner genotype. However, most of these end in miscarriage so the actual proportion of liveborn babies with Turner's syndrome is much lower.

| System | Condition |
|---|---|
| Gastrointestinal | Duodenal atresia<br>Imperforate anus<br>Hirschsprung's disease<br>Coeliac disease |
| Cardiovascular (congenital) | Atrioventricular septal defect (in 40% of patients)<br>Ventricular septal defect (in 30% of patients) |
| Central nervous system | Epilepsy<br>Strabismus<br>Autistic behaviours<br>Alzheimer's disease (early onset) |
| Malignancy | Acute myeloid leukaemia |
| Endocrine | Hypothyroidism |
| Others | Recurrent otitis media<br>Lax ligaments<br>Atlantoaxial instability<br>Decreased fertility<br>Obstructive sleep apnoea |

AVSD, atrioventricular septal defect; VSD, ventricular septal defect.

**Table 14.1** Conditions associated with Down's syndrome

*Clinical features*  The features of Turner's syndrome (**Table 14.3**) are very variable and are similar to those of Noonan's syndrome. Some affected females have a mosaic karyotype (46XX/45XO); they often show a milder form of the syndrome. Not all features need to be present for Turner's syndrome to be diagnosed (**Figure 14.2**).

### Klinefelter's syndrome
Klinefelter's syndrome (46XXY) results when there is an extra X chromosome in a person who is phenotypically male.

## Clinical insight

Hypogonadism is the primary gonadal failure found in both Turner's and Klinefelter's syndromes. It refers to the reduced production of sex hormones and not the size of the sex organs. Although streak ovaries and small testicles can be found in these two conditions, the size is the cause of, and not synonymous with, the hypogonadism.

| Feature | Patau's syndrome | Edwards' syndrome |
|---------|------------------|-------------------|
| Trisomy | Chromosome 13 | Chromosome 18 |
| Head | Microcephaly | Microcephaly<br>Prominent occiput |
| Face | Low-set ears<br>Proboscis<br>Cleft palate<br>Structural eye defects<br>(microphthalmia, coloboma,<br>cyclopia) | Low-set malformed ears<br>Micrognathia<br>Upturned nose<br>Bilateral ptosis<br>Hypertelorism |
| Brain | Holoprosencephaly<br>Optic nerve hypoplasia<br>Global developmental delay | Global developmental delay<br>Choroid plexus cysts |
| Thorax/spine | Meningomyelocoeles | Short sternum |
| Abdomen | Omphalocoele | Oesophageal atresia |
| Heart | Congenital heart defects | Congenital heart defects |
| Limbs | Polydactyly<br>Overlapping digits<br>Rocker-bottom feet | Toe webbing<br>Overlapping digits<br>Rocker-bottom feet |
| Urogenital system | Abnormal genitalia<br>Kidney dysplasia | Undescended testes |
| Prognosis | Mean survival 12 days<br>20% reach 1 year | Mean survival 15 days<br>10% reach 1 year |

**Table 14.2** Features of Edwards' and Patau's syndromes

Symptoms are very often not apparent until boys reach puberty, although there may be a history of mild muscle weakness.

*Clinical features* Klinefelter's syndrome usually manifests as hypogonadism in boys. As a result, during puberty they have broader hips, lower muscle mass, less body hair and more breast tissue (gynaecomastia) than their peers. Despite the reduced testosterone levels, they often grow taller than their peers. They are often infertile.

## Microdeletion syndromes
Microdeletions are regions of genetic material that have broken off chromosomes, leaving them shortened and

| Facial features | Body features |
|---|---|
| Tall forehead | Short stature |
| Downward slanting hypertelorism | Lymphoedema |
| Drooping eyelids | Broad 'shield' chest |
| Low prominent rotated ears | Widely spaced nipples |
| Deep philtrum | Streak-like ovaries |
| Low posterior hairline | Hips and waist of similar width |
| Cystic hygroma | Short fourth metacarpal |
| 'Webbed neck' | Heart defects |
| Crowded teeth | Pubertal delay |

**Table 14.3** Features of Turner's syndrome

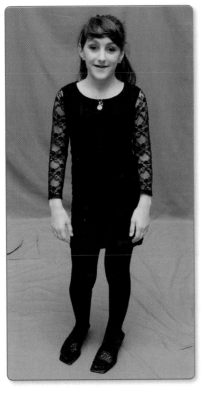

**Figure 14.2** A girl with Turner's syndrome. Note the hypertelorism, low ears, deep philtrum and hip-to-waist ratio. However, the normal neck and chest demonstrates that 'classic signs' are not present in all cases.

incomplete. Many genes may be lost in a single microdeletion. Microdeletions are often 'dominant' in nature, meaning that only one aberrant chromosome is required for pathology to manifest. Some genes on the other copy of the chromosome will be functional, resulting in a very varied spectrum of severity, from severely affected to easily unnoticed.

Microdeletion syndromes are currently diagnosed by fluorescence in situ hybridisation. Four of the most common are:

- 22q microdeletion syndrome
- Williams' syndrome
- Prader–Willi syndrome
- Angelman syndrome

## 22q microdeletion syndrome (including Di George syndrome)

This is is a deletion of genes from the long arm (q) of chromosome 22, most commonly from region 1, band 1.2, in which case it is known as 22q11.2 deletion syndrome. It affects the in utero development of the third and fourth branchial pouches. In 95% of cases, this is a new mutation rather than an inherited condition.

There has been a move away from the name 'DiGeorge syndrome' because this name merely describes a particularly severe subgroup of people with this particular genetic anomaly.

*Clinical features*  The most common feature of 22q microdeletion syndrome is learning difficulties, which may be the first sign in a child whose appearance is normal. The most common dysmorphic features are hypertelorism, micrognathia and low-set ears.

Many cases of 22q microdeletion syndromes are diagnosed late because too much emphasis is placed by clinicians on the mnemonic CATCH-22:

- **C**left palate (feeding difficulties)
- **A**bnormal face (hypertelorism, micrognathia)
- **T**hymic hypoplasia (immunodeficiency)
- **C**ardiac abnormalities (tetralogy of Fallot page 112)
- **H**ypoparathyroidism (hypocalcaemia)
- Chromosome **22**

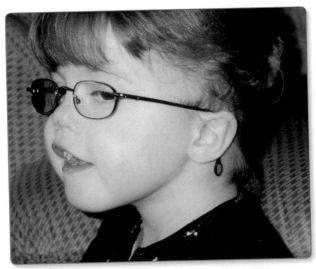

**Figure 14.3** A girl with 22q microdeletion syndrome. Low-set ears and micrognathia are seen here.

This mnemonic should be applied with caution. The majority of children with a 22q microdeletion syndrome do not have immunodeficiency, cleft palates or hypoparathyroidism. The mnemonic stipulates the most severe potential problems caused by the condition, and not the diagnostic criteria.

## Williams' syndrome

Williams' syndrome is caused by a deletion of genes from 7q11.23 – region 1, band 1.23 on the long arm (q) of chromosome 7. This region contains the *ELN* gene, which encodes elastin; among its other functions, this protein allows skin to return to its original shape when stretched.

*Clinical features* Many of the features of Williams' syndrome relate to the poor production of elastin. They include:

- an 'elfin' face (**Figure 14.4**)
- puffy eyes
- a small upturned nose

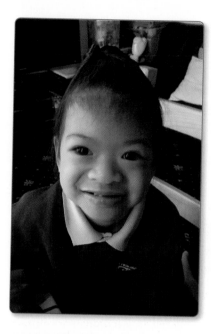

**Figure 14.4** A girl with Williams' syndrome. Note the prominent cheeks, peg-like teeth and wide mouth.

- a wide mouth
- peg-shaped teeth
- hyperacusis
- an overly friendly personality
- learning difficulty
- hypercalcaemia
- cardiac abnormalities (aortic or pulmonary stenosis)

## Prader–Willi and Angelman syndromes

Prader–Willi and Angelman syndromes are caused by a micro-deletion of 15q11–13. The syndrome that manifests depends on whether the aberrant chromosome has been inherited from the mother or the father. This is because of imprinting, an epigenetic phenomenon in which the methylation of different cytosine bases on otherwise normal genes confers different phenotypes.

*Clinical features*  Angelman syndrome (maternally inherited) is characterised by learning difficulties, poor coordination and a classic facies of microcephaly, telecanthus, epicanthic folds and a wide mouth. The combination of a constantly happy demeanour, the facial features and a waddling gait has been uncharitably referred to as a 'happy puppet' appearance.

Prader–Willi syndrome (paternally inherited) is characterised by extreme hyperphagia (uncontrollable eating), but this only starts at around age 2 years. Earlier signs include hypotonia, cryptorchidism, hypogonadism and developmental delay.

## Autosomal dominant syndromes

An autosomal dominant syndrome is one in which the abnormal phenotype (the syndrome) is expressed when there is a mutation in only one of the copies (alleles) of a particular gene. A normal, functioning allele is not able to compensate for the abnormal activity of the mutant copy, which is said to be 'dominant' over it. Autosomal dominant syndromes are either directly inherited from one parent or arise as de novo mutations.

Generally, autosomal dominant syndromes predispose carriers to multiple tumours or produce abnormalities of connective tissue, although there are exceptions, such as Noonan's syndrome (**Table 14.4**).

## X-linked syndromes

Syndromes that derive from genetic aberrations involving the X chromosome manifest with different frequencies in boys and girls:

- X-linked recessive conditions are most common in boys because males do not have a second X chromosome; instead they have a Y chromosome and therefore, unlike girls, cannot be carrying an additional, normal, dominant copy of an allele.
- X-linked dominant conditions are either evenly distributed between the sexes, or are only present in girls if a homozygous state is lethal and a heterozygous state is not.

The two most commonly encountered X-linked dominant syndromes are:

| Syndrome | Features |
|----------|----------|
| **Multiple tumours** | |
| Neurofibromatosis | Café-au-lait spots<br>Subcutaneous growths (neurofibromas)<br>Hamartomas of the iris (Lisch nodules)<br>Scoliosis |
| Tuberous sclerosis | Cerebral and retinal tumours<br>Learning difficulties<br>Tumours of heart and kidney<br>'Ash leaf' hypopigmented macules<br>Citrus-peel pigmented 'shagreen' patches<br>Facial angiofibromas |
| Multiple endocrine neoplasia | Multiple tumours of endocrine organs<br>Symptoms depend on hormones released |
| **Connective tissue disorders** | |
| Marfan's syndrome | Tall habitus with long arms<br>Arachnodactyly<br>Lens dislocation<br>Chest wall abnormalities<br>Scoliosis<br>High-arched palate<br>Heart valve prolapse |
| Ehlers–Danlos syndrome | Joint hypermobility<br>Easy dislocation/subluxation<br>Hyperelastic skin, easy scarring<br>Postural orthostatic tachycardia<br>Bowel obstruction |
| Achondroplasia | Short body<br>Short proximal limbs<br>Sleep apnoea<br>Frontal bossing, narrow foramen magnum<br>Recurrent ear infections |
| Craniosynostosis syndromes (Crouzon's, Apert's, Pfeiffer's) | Fusion of sutures<br>Abnormal skull growth<br>Exophthalmos<br>Hypertelorism<br>Syndactyly<br>Crowded teeth |

**Table 14.4** Autosomal dominant inherited syndromes. *Continues overleaf*

| Other | |
|---|---|
| Noonan's syndrome | Turner-like body habitus<br>Pulmonary stenosis, hypertrophic obstructive cardiomyopathy or septal defect<br>Bleeding disorders<br>Learning difficulties<br>Undescended testes |

**Table 14.4** *Continued*

- fragile X syndrome
- Rett's syndrome

## Fragile X syndrome

The *FMR1* gene is found on the long arm of the X chromosome. The protein for which it codes has a key role in synaptic plasticity – the ability of the brain to alter its neuronal connections. A normal *FMR1* gene contains 4–50 repetitions of the bases CGG. An abnormal number of repetitions of the CGG triplet, especially >200, leads to a reduced production of the FMR protein. This results in fragile X syndrome.

***Clinical features*** The features are often more pronounced in boys than girls, as males do not have a second X chromosome to provide the FMR protein. Key features of fragile X syndrome are:
- long face (**Figure 14.5**)
- protruding ears
- long hyperextendable fingers
- hypotonia
- macro-orchidism
- learning difficulties
- autism or attention deficit hyperactivity disorder behaviours

## Rett's syndrome

Rett's syndrome occurs almost exclusively in girls because boys who carry the *MECP2* gene mutation die in utero or shortly after birth. Rett's syndrome is a neurodevelopmental disorder. Although it sometimes seems to present as neurodegeneration, there is no marked neuronal death in children with the condition.

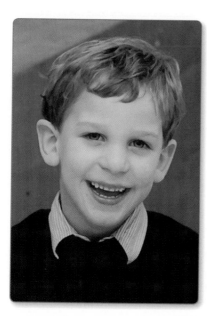

**Figure 14.5** A boy with fragile X syndrome. Note the prominent, large ears and long face shape.

*Clinical features* The classic presentation of Rett's syndrome is a scoliotic girl with autistic behaviours, global developmental delay and hand-wringing stereotypies. Seizure disorders are common. Rett's syndrome progresses in a characteristic manner, as shown in **Table 14.5**.

## Autosomal recessive syndromes

In autosomal recessive syndromes, a mutation in both copies of the gene is required to create an abnormal phenotype. These conditions can occur in the children of asymptomatic heterozygous parents (**Figure 14.6**).

Autosomal recessive conditions cause the loss of a particular enzyme or transport protein. They therefore tend to result in diseases (e.g. sickle cell disease and spinal muscular atrophy) rather than syndromes. Exceptions include

**Clinical insight**

Adult-onset polycystic kidney disease is an autosomal dominant condition, but childhood polycystic kidney disease is autosomal recessive.

| Stage | Name | Age of onset | Features |
|---|---|---|---|
| 0 | Birth | Birth | Apparent normality |
| I | Early onset | 6–18 months | Slowing of head growth<br>Reduced eye contact and interaction<br>Delay in crawling |
| II | Rapid destructive | 1–4 years | Loss of language and purposeful movement<br>Motor stereotypies (hand-wringing, tapping)<br>Irritability<br>Slowing of head growth |
| III | Plateau | 2–10 years | Apraxia<br>Seizures<br>Improvement in behaviours |
| IV | Late motor deterioration | Unspecified | Muscle weakness<br>Spinal curvature<br>Abnormal posturing<br>Spasticity |

Table 14.5 Progression of Rett's syndrome

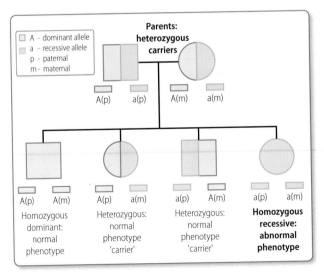

Figure 14.6 Autosomal recessive inheritance.

situs inversus (where the internal organs lie on the opposite side of the body from their anatomical norm).

## Non-genetic syndromes

Many syndromes are not caused by genetic abnormalities but are the result of developmental problems in utero. Examples include:

- fetal alcohol syndrome
- exposure to drugs in utero
- Poland syndrome
- arthrogryposis
- congenital infections

### Fetal alcohol syndrome

Fetal alcohol syndrome is a combination of physical and cognitive features that arise as a result of high maternal alcohol intake during pregnancy.

***Clinical features*** A child with fetal alcohol syndrome (**Figure 14.7**) will have some of the following classic features:

- a history of regular maternal alcohol consumption in pregnancy
- learning difficulties

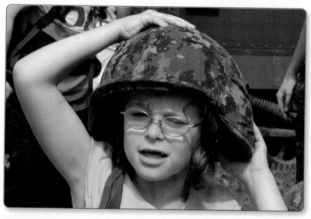

**Figure 14.7** A girl with fetal alcohol syndrome. Note the smooth philtrum and thin upper lip.

- impulsive behaviour
- a thin upper lip
- a smooth philtrum
- a flat midface
- epicanthic folds
- microcephaly
- micrognathia

As with many other syndromes in this chapter, most children with fetal alcohol syndrome will not present with all or even most of the 'classic' features. The most common presentation is impulsive behaviours and learning difficulties, without the classic facial features.

### Teratogenic drugs

Many therapeutic and recreational drugs can cause congenital abnormalities in newborn babies. Examples are listed in **Table 14.6**.

### Poland syndrome

In Poland syndrome, the in utero development of the chest and arm on one side of the body is impeded, resulting in a unilateral absence of the pectoralis muscles. The condition frequently results in malformation of the ribs, arm and hand on the same side. The cause is suspected to be interrupted blood flow during gestation.

### Arthrogryposis

Arthrogryposis is curvature of multiple joints in the developing fetus. It is associated with oligohydramnios (low volumes of amniotic fluid) and reduced fetal movements. The abnormal joint shapes cause congenital muscle fibrosis, resulting in limited movement at the affected joints (**Figure 14.8**).

### Congenital infection syndromes

Congenital infection syndromes result from the antenatal infection of mothers by agents that cause developmental abnormalities. Key examples include cytomegalovirus, rubella virus, Zika virus and *Toxoplasma* (**Table 14.7**).

| Drug | Features |
|------|----------|
| Angiotensin-converting enzyme inhibitors | Renal defects<br>Growth restriction |
| Lithium | Heart valve defects (Ebstein's anomaly) |
| Retinoic acid derivatives (vitamin A) | Malformation of ears |
| Sodium valproate | Neural tube defects<br>Very thin vermillion border to lips<br>Downturned mouth<br>Epicanthic folds<br>Intellectual impairment<br>Radial limb deformity<br>Overlapping digits |
| Tetracyclines and streptomycin | Neural tube defects |
| Thalidomide | Severe limb dysplasia |
| Warfarin | Congenital heart defects<br>Agenesis of corpus callosum,<br>'Stippled epiphyses' on radiography<br>Pectus carinatum<br>Poor growth |
| **Recreational drug** | **Features** |
| Alcohol | Fetal alcohol syndrome (page 300) |
| Benzodiazepines | Neonatal abstinence syndrome |
| Cocaine* | Impaired neurodevelopment<br>Impaired cognition |
| Opiates | Neonatal abstinence syndrome |
| Tobacco | Growth restriction |
| *Cocaine is a potent vasoconstrictor so disrupts blood flow to and within the fetus | |

**Table 14.6** Drugs causing abnormalities of the fetus

## 14.3 Examination for genetic syndromes

When examining a child who appears to have dysmorphic features, describe all the findings carefully and do not try to guess the diagnosis on first inspection. Follow the sequence:

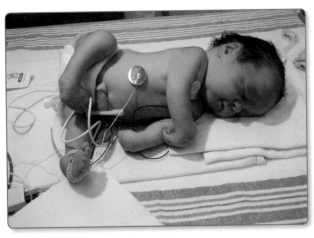

**Figure 14.8** A newborn with arthrogryposis.

- general inspection
- head
- facial features
- chest
- limbs
- genitalia

## General inspection

Stand back and inspect the child, looking particularly at the following:

- Development – does the child have motor or intellectual impairment? Do they walk independently? Are they in a wheelchair or able to mobilise with walking aids?
- Behaviour – does the child show stereotyped behaviours? Are they hyperactive? Are there signs of self-injury?
- Interaction – are the child's social skills normal? Do they make eye contact? Can they converse normally? Do they have social anxiety (see **Chapter 13**)?
- Growth – is the child particularly tall (e.g. Marfan's and Klinefelter's syndromes) or short (e.g. Turner's or Down's syndrome) for their age?

| Maternal infection | Effect on fetus |
|---|---|
| Cytomegalovirus | Low birthweight<br>Microcephaly<br>Petechiae<br>Hepatomegaly with jaundice<br>Sensorineural deafness<br>Learning difficulties |
| Rubella | Sensorineural deafness<br>Microphthalmia<br>Cataract<br>Pulmonary artery stenosis<br>'Blueberry muffin' rash*<br>Global developmental delay |
| Toxoplasma | Micro- or macrocephaly<br>Hydrocephalus<br>Cerebral calcium deposits<br>Global developmental delay<br>Sensory impairments<br>Hepatosplenomegaly<br>Lymphadenopathy |
| Zika virus | Microcephaly<br>Abnormal brain development<br>Global developmental delay<br>Retinal damage<br>Spasticity<br>Limb contractures |

*Non-blanching rash caused by thrombocytopenia and extramedullary haematopoiesis.

Table 14.7 Syndromes caused by antenatal infections

- Proportion – is the child's growth in proportion? Do they have a large head but shortened limbs, as in achondroplasia?
- Family members – does the child look like a relative who has previously been investigated for any similar appearance or congenital abnormality?

## Head

Assess the size and shape of the head. In younger children, check the sutures and fontanelles for closure.

| Microcephaly | Macrocephaly |
|---|---|
| Genetic syndromes<br>Prenatal infection<br>Prenatal ischaemia<br>Craniosynostosis (premature fusion of the sutures) | Hydrocephalus<br>Fragile X syndrome<br>Overgrowth conditions, e.g.<br>Beckwith-Weideman syndrome |

Table 14.8 Non-idiopathic causes of abnormal head size

First, use a tape to measure the maximum occipitofrontal circumference. Plot this on a centile chart.

Next:

- check whether the anterior fontanelle is open and, if so, whether it is bulging or sunken
- feel along the skull sutures for abnormalities (early or late fusion, ridges or abnormal shapes)
- look for bossing (**Figure 14.10**), a protuberance of the frontal bones, which is congenital (for example in achondroplasia) or acquired (in rickets and beta thalassaemia)

**Figure 14.9** shows the sutures and fontanelles of the infant skull.

> ## Clinical insight
>
> Microcephaly is defined as an occipitofrontal circumference below the 0.4th centile. Macrocephaly is defined as an occipitofrontal circumference above the 99.6th centile. Both can be normal findings, particularly if there is a family history of this, but both can also suggest particular clinical syndromes (Table 14.8).

**Appearance** One side of the skull can be flattened (plagiocephaly, **Figure 14.10**). This may be:

- benign deformational plagiocephaly, a simple mechanical issue arising from the child lying preferentially with their head to one side
- benign deformational brachycephaly (**Figure 14.10**), a flattened occiput that arises from lying preferentially with their head straight
- unilateral craniosynostosis – premature closure of one of the sutures

**Associated conditions** Craniosynostosis syndromes include Apert's, Crouzon's and Pfeiffer's syndromes, which are described in **Table 14.4**.

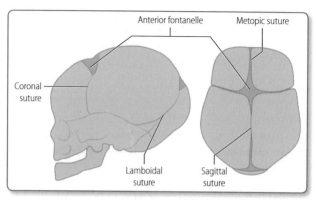

**Figure 14.9** Normal sutures of the infant skull.

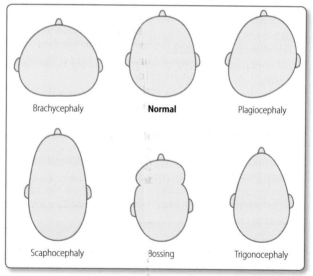

**Figure 14.10** Abnormal head shapes.

The most common forms of craniosynostosis are:

- sagittal synostosis – premature fusion of the sagittal suture resulting in a narrow elongated head, which is called scapho-cephaly (**Figure 14.10**)
- coronal synostosis – premature fusion of the coronal suture; if bilateral, this results in a tall pointed head shape called turricephaly
- metopic synostosis – premature fusion of the metopic suture, between the two frontal bones, resulting in a trian-gular shaped head called trigonocephaly (**Figure 14.10**).

## Face

If a child is dysmorphic, it is important to be able to describe the face with precision in order to come to an accurate diagnosis.

## Eyes

The following should be noted:

- What are the interpupillary and intercanthic distances (**Figure 14.11**)? Hypertelorism describes orbits that are unusually far apart. Telecanthus is when the eye is partially covered by a widened medial canthus
- Do the eyelids droop (bilateral ptosis)?
- Are the folds of skin at the inner aspect of the eye prominent (epicanthic folds)?
- Do the palpebral fissures slant upwards (e.g. in Down's syn-drome) or downwards (e.g. in Noonan's syndrome)?
- Look for defects in the iris (coloboma ) and for the star-shaped (stellate) iris characteristic of Williams' syndrome (see page 293).

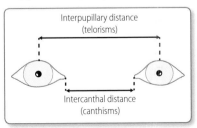

**Figure 14.11**
Measurement of eye spacing.

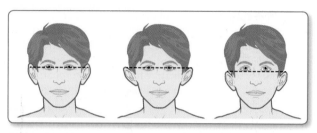

**Figure 14.12** Measurement of ear position. (a) Normal position. (b) Normal position masked by the angle of the pinna. (c) Low-set ears.

## Ears

Examine the ears for:
- size and shape (large ears are seen in fragile X syndrome)
- position (low-set ears can be seen in all karyotype disorders and 22q microdeletion syndrome)
- pre- and post-auricular skin tags

Low-set ears must be distinguished from normally set ears that are unusually angled. To judge the setting of the ears, picture a horizontal plane through the canthi. The helix of the ear should meet the skull above this line (**Figure 14.12**).

## Mouth, nose and philtrum

Inspect the mouth for:
- cleft lip and/or palate, which can be an isolated feature or linked with 22q microdeletion syndrome
- the shape of the mouth and tongue – a small mouth and large tongue are found in Down's syndrome
- the philtrum, the groove that connects the mouth to the nose – a smooth philtrum is seen in fetal alcohol syndrome
- the teeth, which are spiked in Williams' syndrome

## Thorax

Examine the chest for:
- shape – it may be barrel-shaped or shield-shaped, or demonstrate pectus excavatum or pectus carinatum
- musculature, which may be absent in Poland syndrome (see page 301)

- pubertal development, to assess Tanner staging in girls (see Chapter 4)
- webbing of the neck, seen in Turner's and Noonan's syndromes

Also look at the spine, which may show signs of scoliosis (see Chapter 10).

Always complete a full cardiovascular examination (see **Chapter 7**) when considering a genetic syndrome. This is because many syndromes are associated with congenital heart disease so murmurs will be heard.

## Limbs

Examine the limbs, looking for:

- asymmetry
- abnormal length (e.g. short limbs in achondroplasia)
- abnormal shape (e.g. rocker-bottom feet in Edward's syndrome)
- abnormal tone or flexibility
- polydactyly and syndactyly
- clinodactyly (shortened digits)
- positioning of the limbs (e.g. talipes)
- single palmar creases

## Genitalia

Examine the genitalia for evidence of:

- ambiguous genitalia
- Tanner staging (puberty may be delayed in Turner's syndrome)
- testicular size, which may be increased (e.g. in fragile X syndrome) or decreased (e.g. in Klinefelter's syndrome).

> ## Clinical insight
>
> Do not place too much emphasis on any single physical finding. For example, 50% of children with Down's syndrome do not have a single palmar crease, and most single palmar creases are benign and idiopathic.

## Finishing the examination

Dysmorphia is often a sign of a wider genetic syndrome, which may affect multiple organ systems. If you are confident in the observation of dysmorphic features, then ensure that the following are all documented:

- growth examination (Chapter 4)
- development examination (Chapter 5)
- respiratory examination (Chapter 6)
- cardiac examination (Chapter 7)
- abdominal examination (Chapter 8)
- neurological examination (Chapter 9)
- musculoskeletal examination (Chapter 10)
- ENT examination (Chapter 11)
- skin examination (Chapter 12)
- behavioural assessment (Chapter 13)

## 14.4 Examination summary

A summary of how to examine a child for features of multisystem syndromes is given in **Table 14.9**.

| Component | Key findings |
|---|---|
| General inspection | Abnormal growth, development, behaviour |
| Head | Skull shape, circumference, fused sutures, asymmetry |
| Face | Eye setting, coloboma, epicanthic folds, ptosis, ear setting, philtrum, mouth shape, dentition |
| Chest | Heart murmur, chest shape, neck webbing, Tanner staging (girls) |
| Limbs | Limb shape, digits, palmar creases, arthrogryposis |
| Genitalia | Undescended testes, ambiguous genitalia, Tanner staging (boys) |
| Investigations | Karyotype, fluorescence in situ hybridisation, echocardiogram, syndrome-specific blood tests or exome/whole genome sequencing |
| Have you ruled out … ? | Risk of malignancy, risk of immunodeficiency, infertility, risk to future siblings |

**Table 14.9** Summary of paediatric syndromic examination and associated investigations

# Index

Note: Page numbers in **bold** or *italic* refer to tables or figures respectively.